Practice Management

Editor

MICHELLE ANNE BHOLAT

PRIMARY CARE:
CLINICS IN OFFICE PRACTICE

www.primarycare.theclinics.com

Consulting Editor
JOEL J. HEIDELBAUGH

December 2012 • Volume 39 • Number 4

ELSEVIER

1600 John F. Kennedy Boulevard, Suite 1800 • Philadelphia, PA 19103-2899

http://www.theclinics.com

PRIMARY CARE: CLINICS IN OFFICE PRACTICE Volume 39, Number 4
December 2012 ISSN 0095-4543, ISBN-13: 978-1-4557-4935-5

Editor: Yonah Korngold

Primary Care: Clinics in Office Practice (ISSN: 0095–4543) is published quarterly by Elsevier Inc., 360 Park Avenue South, New York, NY 10010-1710. Months of issue are March, June, September, and December. Periodicals postage paid at New York, NY and additional mailing offices. Subscription prices are $216.00 per year (US individuals), $353.00 (US institutions), $108.00 (US students), $264.00 (Canadian individuals), $415.00 (Canadian institutions), $169.00 (Canadian students), $329.00 (international individuals), $415.00 (international institutions), and $169.00 (international students). Foreign air speed delivery is included in all *Clinics* subscription prices. All prices are subject to change without notice. POSTMASTER: Send address changes to *Primary Care: Clinics in Office Practice*, Elsevier Periodicals Customer Service, 11830 Westline Industrial Drive, St. Louis, MO 63146. Customer Service Health Sciences Division, Subscription Customer Service, 3251 Riverport Lane, Maryland Heights, MO 63043. **Customer Service: 1-800-654-2452 (U.S. and Canada); 314-447-8871 (outside U.S. and Canada). Fax: 314-447-8029. E-mail: journalscustomerservice-usa@elsevier.com (for print support); journalsonlinesupport-usa@elsevier.com (for online support).**

Reprints. For copies of 100 or more, of articles in this publication, please contact the Commercial Reprints Department, Elsevier Inc., 360 Park Avenue South, New York, NY 10010-1710. Tel. (212) 633-3812; Fax: (212) 482-1935; E-mail: reprints@elsevier.com.

Primary Care: Clinics in Office Practice is covered in *MEDLINE/PubMed (Index Medicus)* and *EMBASE/ Excerpta Medica, Current Contents/Clinical Medicine, and ISI/BIOMED.*

Contributors

CONSULTING EDITOR

JOEL J. HEIDELBAUGH, MD, FAAFP, FACG
Clinirtments of Family Medicine and Urocal Associate Professor, Depalogy, Clerkship Director, Department of Family Medicine, University of Michigan Medical School, Ann Arbor, Michigan; Ypsilanti Health Center, Ypsilanti, Michigan

GUEST EDITOR

MICHELLE ANNE BHOLAT, MD, MPH
Executive Vice Chair, Department of Family Medicine, David Geffen School of Medicine at UCLA, UCLA Family Health Center, Santa Monica, California

AUTHORS

MICHELLE ANNE BHOLAT, MD, MPH
Executive Vice Chair, Department of Family Medicine, David Geffen School of Medicine at UCLA, UCLA Family Health Center, Santa Monica, California

MATTHEW BRENSILVER, PhD
Postdoctoral Fellow, Department of Family Medicine, David Geffen School of Medicine at UCLA, UCLA Family Health Center, Santa Monica, California

BILL DACEY, MHA, MBA, CPC, CPC-I
President, The Dacey Group, Inc, Palm Harbor, Florida

ANAHITA DASHTAEI, PharmD
Sharp Community Pharmacy, Coronado, California

PATRICK T. DOWLING, MD, MPH
Department of Family Medicine, David Geffen School of Medicine at UCLA, Los Angeles, California

BARBARA L. INGRAM, PhD
Professor, Department of Psychology, Graduate School of Education and Psychology, Pepperdine University, Los Angeles, California

BERNARD J. KATZ, MD, MBA
Assistant Professor of Family Medicine, University of California, Los Angeles, Culver City, California

ADABEL LEE, PhD
Assistant Research Psychologist, Global Center for Children and Families, Semel Institute for Neuroscience and Human Behavior, University of California at Los Angeles, Los Angeles, California

SOKKIM LIM, PharmD
Cal eConnect, Inc, Emeryville, California

KIMBERLY LING, PhD
UCLA Family Health Center, Santa Monica, California

MARK R. NEEDHAM, MD, MBA
Assistant Professor of Family Medicine, University of California, Los Angeles, Culver City, California

TINA NGUYEN, PharmD
City of Hope National Medical Center, Duarte, California

LARA RAY, PhD
UCLA Family Health Center, Santa Monica, California

ALISON RETA, PharmD
University of Southern California School of Pharmacy, Los Angeles, California

MARY JANE ROTHERAM-BORUS, PhD
Director, Global Center for Children and Families; Bat-Yaacov Professor of Child Psychiatry and Biobehavioral Sciences, Semel Institute for Neuroscience and Human Behavior, University of California at Los Angeles, Los Angeles, California

STEVEN SHOPTAW, PhD
Professor and Vice Chair, Department of Family Medicine, David Geffen School of Medicine at UCLA, UCLA Family Health Center, Santa Monica, California

LYNN STEPHENS, FN, FNP, MN
Family Nurse Practitioner, Department of Family Medicine, David Geffen School of Medicine at UCLA, Santa Monica, California

DALLAS SWENDEMAN, PhD
Co-Director, Global Center for Children and Families; Assistant Professor, Semel Institute for Neuroscience and Human Behavior, University of California at Los Angeles, Los Angeles, California

SHABANA TARIQ, MD
Postdoctoral Fellow, Department of Family Medicine, David Geffen School of Medicine at UCLA, California

DAVID J. WALLENSTEIN, MD
Associate Clinical Professor, Director, Family Medicine Outpatient Pain and Palliative Care Clinic; Department of Family Medicine, University of California at Los Angeles, Los Angeles, California

Contents

Foreword: The Playbook for Primary Care Practice Management　　　　ix

Joel J. Heidelbaugh

Preface　　　　xi

Michelle Anne Bholat

Family Nurse Practitioners: "Value Add" in Outpatient Chronic Disease Management　　　595

Lynn Stephens

> Nurse practitioners are capable leaders in primary care design as practices nationwide move to consider and adopt the patient-centered medical home. The chronic care model provides a structure to enhance the care of chronic illness. Nurse practitioners are instrumental in many areas of this model as both leaders and caregivers. Safety and quality are basic medical home goals; nurse practitioners enhance both. The addition of a nurse practitioner to a practice is an effective "value add" in every way.

Integration of Behavioral Medicine in Primary Care　　　605

Michelle Anne Bholat, Lara Ray, Matthew Brensilver, Kimberly Ling, and Steven Shoptaw

> The health care system in the United States is inefficient and there are many incentives for sustainable changes in the delivery of care. Incorporating behavioral medicine offers a wide range of opportunities. Within primary care settings, pain disorders, addiction, depression, and anxiety disorders are highly prevalent. Numerous chronic health conditions also require behavioral support for lifestyle change. These disorders are optimally managed through interdisciplinary collaborations that include a behavioral medicine component. This article discusses the effective integration of behavioral medicine within a primary care patient-centered medical home and describes the organizational planning and structure required for success.

Opportunities to Improve Clinical Outcomes and Challenges to Implementing Clinical Pharmacists into Health Care Teams　　　615

Alison Reta, Anahita Dashtaei, Sokkim Lim, Tina Nguyen, and Michelle Anne Bholat

> Improving patient care outcomes is achieved through communication, collaboration, and coordination of care between various health care professionals in all health care practice settings. The foundation of this patient-centered model approach includes the recognition of pharmacists as drug therapy experts and, therefore, as members of the health care team who provide a unique set of knowledge and skills. This article focuses on improving clinical outcomes by integrating clinical pharmacists into health care teams, and addresses the obstacles and solutions to achieving this goal.

Palliative Care in the Patient-Centered Medical Home   627

David J. Wallenstein

There are few published data on the delivery of palliative care services in the outpatient setting and virtually none on either the integration of palliative care into primary care practice or its applicability to innovative models of health care delivery, such as the patient-centered medical home and accountable care organizations. In this article, new topics for health services delivery research are suggested. Because of the lack of data, the article draws on information collected from inpatient palliative care delivery and includes anecdotal experiences from the outpatient pain medicine and palliative care clinic of an academic department of family medicine.

Health Information Technology: Medical Record Documentation Issues in the Electronic Era   633

Bill Dacey and Michelle Anne Bholat

This article outlines the regulatory movement propelling physicians into the electronic health record environment and the subsequent emergence of quality issues in the medical record. There are benefits and downside risks for implementing electronic health records as part of the desire of a practice or institution to build patient-centered medical homes. The intersection of how a practice or institution collects and reports quality metrics using health information technology and subsequently submits claims for services rendered has created unforeseen challenges for which leadership must be aware and address proactively.

Utilizing International Medical Graduates in Health Care Delivery: Brain Drain, Brain Gain, or Brain Waste? A Win-Win Approach at University of California, Los Angeles   643

Patrick T. Dowling and Michelle Anne Bholat

After identifying many unlicensed Hispanic international medical graduates (IMGs) legally residing in southern California, University of California, Los Angeles developed an innovative program to prepare these sidelined physicians to enter family medicine residency programs and become licensed physicians. On completion of a 3-year family medicine residency-training program, these IMGs have an obligation to practice in a federally designated underserved community in the state for 2 to 3 years. As the US health care system moves from physician-centered practices to patient-focused teams, with primary care serving as the foundation for building patient-centered medical homes, attention to educating IMGs in these concepts is crucial.

Adoption of Self-Management Interventions for Prevention and Care   649

Mary Jane Rotheram-Borus, Barbara L. Ingram, Dallas Swendeman, and Adabel Lee

Seventy-five percent of health care costs can be attributed to chronic diseases, making prevention and management imperative. Collaborative patient self-management in primary care is efficacious in reducing symptoms and increasing quality of life. In this article, the authors argue that self-management interventions span the continuum of prevention and disease management. Self-management interventions rest on a foundation of 5 core actions: (1) activate motivation to change, (2) apply domain-specific information from education and self-monitoring, (3) develop skills, (4) acquire environmental resources, and (5) build social support. Several delivery vehicles are described and evaluated in terms of diffusion and cost-containment goals.

Optimizing Pain Management Through Collaborations with Behavioral and Addiction Medicine in Primary Care   661

Matthew Brensilver, Shabana Tariq, and Steven Shoptaw

Chronic noncancer pain (CNCP) affects many primary care patients, and carries a large human and economic burden. In response to the widespread perception that pain is underdiagnosed and undertreated, regulatory bodies have encouraged more comprehensive services to address pain syndromes. Significant hurdles exist in treating CNCP in primary care settings, and interventional therapies and pharmacotherapy often do not provide complete symptomatic relief. This article describes a multidimensional and interdisciplinary approach to the treatment of CNCP. The utility of collaborations with behavioral and addiction medicine specialists optimizes care and advances models of patient treatment within a primary care patient-centered medical home.

Bending the Cost Curve and Increasing Revenue: A Family Medicine Model that Works!   671

Bernard J. Katz and Mark R. Needham

This article attempts to illustrate ways in which family physician practices are able to demonstrate high value, enhanced quality, and streamlined costs, essential components of practice sustainability. Specific examples are provided to assist practices to consider questions and information that allow for skillful engagement during contract negotiations, consider increasing practice revenues by adopting practice enhancements that make sense for the location of the practice and community needs, develop workflow analyses, and review opportunities for expense reduction.

Index   683

PRIMARY CARE:
CLINICS IN OFFICE PRACTICE

FORTHCOMING ISSUE

March 2013
Cardiovascular Disease
Robert Sheeler, MD, *Guest Editor*

RECENT ISSUES

September 2012
Low Back Pain
Eron Manusov, MD, *Guest Editor*

June 2012
Chronic Disease Management
Brooke Salzman, MD,
Lauren Collins, MD, and
Emily R. Hajjar, PharmD, *Guest Editors*

March 2012
Prenatal Care
David R. Harnisch Sr, MD,
Guest Editor

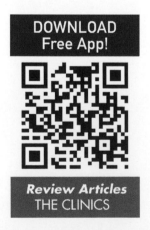

Foreword

The Playbook for Primary Care Practice Management

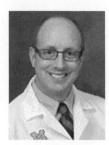

Joel J. Heidelbaugh, MD, FAAFP, FACG
Consulting Editor

In reading the articles for this volume of *Primary Care: Clinics in Office Practice* dedicated to practice management, I became nostalgic thinking about when I was applying to medical school. As for most applicants, colleges and universities require a personal statement of some form where we highlight our passions for entering the field of medicine. Then, there is a usually an interview process with a panel of professors dubbed the "Pre-Professional Advisory Committee," or some other very similar moniker. In 1991, when I was invited to discuss my dreams of becoming a physician and convince the committee that I was a suitable candidate for admission to medical school, I was asked, "what will be the greatest challenge facing physicians in the coming years"?

My answer was both insightful and foreshadowing: "the physician of the future will not only need to be adept at medical science and current in knowledge with new medications, therapies, and technologies, but will also require a keen understanding of the business aspects of medicine with respect to cost-effective provisions of care and integration between various levels of providers." Not realizing that my answer would serve as the proverbial "lightning rod," a member of the committee retorted, "I recommend that this committee NOT support your application to medical school, because medicine is a science, NOT a business!" Hanging my head low, I figured I had blown my chances for endorsement as a medical school applicant. Perhaps not ironically, we ALL now recognize that medicine, for better or for worse, is an exceptionally complicated business paradigm, and a national crisis requiring the need for immediate and powerful reform due to rapidly escalating costs.

In this volume of *Primary Care: Clinics in Office Practice*, impressively the topics of utilizing international medical graduates and integrating behavioral medicine, palliative care, and pain management in primary care offer guidelines for augmenting our daily practices. Every aspect of practice management is now dependent on electronic medical records, as most practices and clinicians use some form of this on a daily basis; yet, the challenges of ensuring adequate and appropriate documentation to

Prim Care Clin Office Pract 39 (2012) ix–x
http://dx.doi.org/10.1016/j.pop.2012.09.001 **primarycare.theclinics.com**

capture revenue and meet meaningful use criteria loom with great importance. Articles dedicated to providing salient information on improving clinical outcomes in chronic disease management with the alliance of pharmacists and nurse practitioners provide invaluable details that most of us haven't been formally taught, but which are imperative to daily practice.

Perhaps most notable is a very forward-thinking article entitled, "Bending the Cost Curve and Increasing Revenue: A Family Medicine Model that Works." As primary care practices continue to feel short-changed for they complexity of care that they provide (and the associated administrative responsibilities…), this article offers innovative suggestions for marrying complex care management to both improve outcomes and decrease costs.

I thank Dr Michelle Bholat, Vice Chair in the Department of Family Medicine at UCLA, and her colleagues for their very comprehensive and informative compilation of articles in this volume of *Primary Care: Clinics in Office Practice*, as I know that we will all gain additional useful knowledge across various aspects of practice management that we can use and teach in our daily practices.

Joel J. Heidelbaugh, MD, FAAFP, FACG
Departments of Family Medicine and Urology
University of Michigan Medical School
Ann Arbor, MI 48109, USA

Ypsilanti Health Center
200 Arnet Street, Suite 200
Ypsilanti, MI 48198, USA

E-mail address:
jheidel@umich.edu

Preface

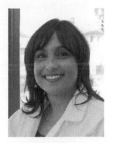

Michelle Anne Bholat, MD, MPH
Guest Editor

I completed my Family Medicine residency and fellowship at a public academic institution in Los Angeles, California, after which I honed my skills in health care and population management at the UCLA School of Public Health. After receiving a Master's degree in Public Health, I had the opportunity to work for The Joint Commission, formerly the Joint Commission on Accreditation of Healthcare Organizations and observe and report on how well government and nongovernment organizations of all sizes and complexities went about the business of delivering safe, high-quality patient care. In addition to broadening my knowledge of US health care, I have traveled internationally working with US AID and most recently with colleagues in South Africa—each challenged with meeting the Institute for Healthcare Improvement's http://www.IHI.org *Triple Aim*. This concept has been eloquently summarized on numerous occasions by former CMS Director Don Berewick as providing, "better care, better health at lower cost." I have the privilege of working with 2 exceptional leaders: A. Eugene Washington, MD, MSc, Vice Chancellor UCLA Health Sciences and Dean of the David Geffen School of Medicine at UCLA, and David Feinberg, MD, MBA, President, UCLA Health System, who are changing how we approach health care, research, education, and community engagement.

The UCLA Department of Family Medicine has a broad mission reflective of the specialty of Family Medicine—caring for individuals from the cradle to the grave. Patrick T. Dowling, MD, MPH, Chair of the Department, has assembled an exceptional group of faculty, many of whom are leaders and innovators in the science of health care delivery, Addiction and Behavioral Medicine, Chronic Disease Management, and Hospice and Palliative Medicine. The UCLA Family Health Center serves as a multidisciplinary innovation center that continues to build on work that began in 2006, utilizing Dr Ed Wagner's Chronic Care Model. The clinic is actively engaged with UCLA Health System Practice Re-design and Ambulatory Operational Excellence efforts under the leadership of Patricia A. Kapur, MD, CEO, UCLA Faculty Practice Group, and Executive VP, UCLA Health System, Molly J. Coye, MD, MPH, Chief Innovation Officer, and Samuel A. Skootsky, MD, Chief Medical Officer Faculty Practice Group and Medical Group.

Although there are many challenges, equally there are opportunities to provide cost-effective, efficient health care to individuals and communities. Whether

Prim Care Clin Office Pract 39 (2012) xi–xiii
http://dx.doi.org/10.1016/j.pop.2012.10.001
0095-4543/12/$ – see front matter © 2012 Published by Elsevier Inc.
primarycare.theclinics.com

reorganization occurs within a practice, clinic, health system, or region, redesign efforts must be coupled with changes in payment. Further, as a nation, we must critically evaluate whether we are developing an adequate number of the type of professionals with the necessary skills to lead twenty-first century health care. Just as new models of health care delivery are emerging, so must new models in education.

The articles in this special edition of *Primary Care: Clinics in Office Practice* brought together a group of professional and research scientist colleagues with expertise and interest to achieve the *Triple Aim*—to provide better care, to achieve better health outcomes, and to do so at lower cost. The authors and topics were selected because they represent cutting-edge ideas and programs for the development or refinement of Patient-Centered Medical Homes (PCMHs). The topics were selected to address the notion of how we view health care delivery based on a model with Hospice and Palliative care at the top of a model pyramid with self-care and wellness at the base.

The apex of the pyramid represents care provided to those nearing the end of life. In Dr Wallenstein's article, "Palliative Care in the *Patient-Centered Medical Home*," he distinguishes hospice from palliative care and notes the paucity of literature regarding the impact of outpatient palliative care on quality and total cost of care. Innovative models for high touch care will emerge as the PCMH Model evolves outside of hospitals and clinics.

The foundation or base of our topical pyramid takes into account that not everyone has a chronic illness. Dr Rotheram and his team assert that self-management interventions can effectively span the continuum of prevention and disease management and explain self-management interventions in terms of diffusion and cost-containment goals in the article, "Adoption of Self-Management Interventions for Prevention and Care." Above the wellness base, 2 articles lend themselves to rethinking addiction as a chronic condition, provide insights to understanding the role of Behavioral Medicine within a primary care practice, and explore the treatment of chronic nonmalignant pain utilizing a multidisciplinary approach. Dr Brensilver addresses these ideas in his article, "Optimizing Pain Management Through Collaborations with Behavioral and Addiction Medicine in Primary Care," while Bholat, Ray, Brensilver, Ling, and Shoptaw shed light on developing a new Behavioral Medicine model of care and provide lessons learned in doing so in their article, "Integration of Behavioral Medicine in Primary Care."

Two additional articles, layered upon the last, focus on improving the treatment and outcomes for patients with chronic conditions. Stephens, in her article, "Family Nurse Practitioners—'Value Add' in Outpatient Chronic Disease Management" describes the role of advanced practice nurses beyond the 1 patient in the examination room at a time model, while the article, "Opportunities to Improve Clinical Outcomes and Challenges to Implementing Clinical Pharmacists into Healthcare Team," Dashtaei, Lim, Nguyen, and colleagues describe the role of the clinical pharmacist within a primary care setting. Because many physicians may not have trained directly with clinical pharmacists, faculty, fellows, residents, and medical students are realizing the value of working side by side a medication specialist.

Also included in this issue are 3 articles that contribute to the next to the last level of the pyramid. Katz and Needham offer readers the opportunity to learn how to create a sustainable practice in their article, "Bending the Cost Curve and Increasing Revenue: A Family Medicine Model That Works!" Linked to revenue enhancement is the use of Health Information Technology (HIT). HIT drives systems to improve individual and population health. According to Dacey, "there is a bit of a dark side to this technology," particularly for the physicians and trainees utilizing the EHR to both collect and report on the specific care provided on a specific day to a patient and subsequently bill for these services. The article, "Health Information Technology: Medical Record Documentation Issues in the Electronic Era," will help administrators and clinicians avoid common and potentially costly errors. The third article addresses international medical graduates (IMGs). IMGs represent 25% of the US physician workforce and are an innovative model as described by Dowling and Bholat in "Utilizing International Medical Graduates in Health Care Delivery: Brain Drain, Brain Gain, or Brain Waste? A Win-Win Approach at UCLA." This program increases the number IMGs who will become family physicians and provides educational opportunities to teach and model the concepts of the PCMH during this preresidency training program.

Michelle Anne Bholat, MD, MPH
Department of Family Medicine
David Geffen School of Medicine at UCLA
UCLA Family Health Center
1920 Colorado Avenue
Santa Monica, CA 90404, USA

E-mail address:
mbholat@mednet.ucla.edu

Family Nurse Practitioners
"Value Add" in Outpatient Chronic Disease Management

Lynn Stephens, FN, FNP, MN

KEYWORDS

- Nurse practitioner • Outpatients • Patient-centered medical home
- Chronic Care Model

KEY POINTS

- As advanced practice nurses, nurse practitioners have a unique skill set. Their basic nursing knowledge provides the foundation for patient-centered care. The additional diagnosis and treatment skills create competency in health maintenance, acute care, and chronic disease management.
- Nurse practitioners are capable leaders in primary care design as practices nationwide move to consider/adopt the patient-centered medical home.
- The chronic care model provides a structure to enhance the care of chronic illness. Nurse practitioners are instrumental in many areas of this model as both leaders and caregivers. Safety and quality are basic medical home goals; nurse practitioners enhance both.

INTRODUCTION

Family nurse practitioners (FNPs) possess a unique skill set that can address all aspects of chronic disease management. There is more than a simple semantic difference between illness and disease. Illness is how the disease is interpreted and managed within a person's life. Nurses are trained to care for the whole person, encompassing the bio-psycho-social-spiritual components of a human being. Nursing addresses the fundamental issues of patient education, adherence, support, and follow-up. Nurse practitioners blend both nursing theory and education, caring for the whole person, with the additional knowledge of disease diagnosis and management.

NURSE PRACTITIONERS

Nurse practitioners are advanced practice nurses whose colleagues are nurse midwives, nurse anesthetists, clinical nurse specialists and nurse executives. The

Conflicts of interest: The author reports no conflicts of interest.
Department of Family Medicine, David Geffen School of Medicine at UCLA, 1920 Colorado Avenue, Santa Monica, CA 90095, USA
E-mail address: lmstephens@mednet.ucla.edu

role of nurse practitioner was developed in 1965. Initially trained in the specialties of family medicine and pediatrics to practice in the outpatient setting, nurse practitioners are specialized in as many different settings as physicians. There are more than 150,000 nurse practitioners in the United States today. According to the American Academy of Nurse Practitioners, about 48% of nurse practitioners are FNPs in outpatient settings and 19.3% work as adult nurse practitioners.[1]

Nurse practitioners have been labeled mid-level providers or physician extenders by the health care system. More accurately, nurse practitioners are high-level, Master's or Doctoral-level trained nurses, not simply mid-level providers of care.[2] A physician extender is an appropriate term for a physician assistant (PA). PAs differ from nurse practitioners in their undergraduate emphasis and subsequent PA training.

EDUCATION

Nurse practitioners graduate with a baccalaureate degree in nursing (BSN). The undergraduate training emphasizes the basic core sciences: anatomy, physiology, chemistry, pathophysiology, and pharmacology. Nursing theory teaches assessment and planning of nursing care that addresses a more complete, in-depth view of the patient as an individual. Nurses are taught to focus on each patient as a unique entity, with their own strengths, weaknesses, coping strategies, culture, language, and education that create a combined impact to their response to an illness. Nurse practitioners have 2 additional years of education to complete a Master's degree in nursing. This additional education is heavily focused on acute and chronic disease management with more advanced pharmacology courses and, typically, outpatient clinical rotations. Clinical professors at Schools of Nursing at the graduate level build on the principles students have learned in undergraduate nursing schools. Fundamental nursing theories of caring for the whole person are crucial in providing safe, effective, quality care.

THE PATIENT-CENTERED MEDICAL HOME

The patient-centered medical home (PCMH), although not a new concept, has gained prominence in the health care industry as a means to provide high-quality and simultaneously lower costs. The following are examples of how 2 national organizations define this concept of care.

National Committee for Quality Assurance

The Patient-Centered Medical Home is a health care setting that facilitates partnerships between individual patients and their personal physicians, and when appropriate, the patient's family. Care is facilitated by registries, information technology, health information exchange, and other means to assure that patients get the indicated care when and where they need and want it in a culturally and linguistically appropriate manner.[3]

American Academy of Family Physicians

A patient-centered medical home integrates patients as active participants in their own health and well-being. Patients are cared for by a physician who leads the medical team that coordinates all aspects of preventive, acute, and chronic needs of patients using the best available evidence and appropriate technology. These relationships offer patients comfort, convenience, and optimal health throughout their lifetimes.[4,5]

These 2 national organizations use words and concepts from the nursing theories of patient participation and patient-centered care. Nurses have been trained to routinely incorporate these concepts in their care, and strive to partner with their patients because trust is the foundation of all caring relationships. Nurses involve the patient and family in the planning of care because people have to be approached as individuals and their personal situations can vary widely. Nursing care plans have outlined "self-management" and have helped patients set goals for their care decades before it became fashionable in the medical literature. What is so exciting is that the medical profession and indeed the health care industry are embracing important nursing theory and putting this into practice.

Nurses seek to work with their patients as problem-solvers and collaborators. While the above definitions state that the physician is the leader of the medical team; the FNP can also serve in this function. Using an FNP to coordinate care, manage a registry of patients, and teach and manage a core of medical assistants and community health coaches, alongside the ability to provide direct patient care, is an important "value add" to busy primary care practices.

THE CHRONIC CARE MODEL

The Chronic Care Model (CCM) was developed by Ed Wagner, MD, MPH and published in 1998. In collaboration with the Institute for Chronic Illness Care, the model was updated in 2003. The purpose of the update to the original CCM was to reflect advances in chronic care both from the research literature and from the scores of health care systems that implemented the Model in their improvement efforts.[6]

As participants in the California Academic Chronic Care Collaborative (2006–2008), the author's academic medical center's teaching family health center was 1 of 19 California residency training programs selected to implement the CCM model.[6] The CCM model of 6 elements was used as a framework for the FNP-led chronic disease medical clinic. These 6 elements include: (1) health care organization support, (2) clinic information systems, (3) self-management, (4) community involvement, (5) decision support, and (6) delivery system design.[7,8] The theory behind the model is to promote positive interactions between a prepared, proactive patient and the health care team as a means to manage chronic disease. The CCM provided the framework needed to create teams and tools to provide better care.

Components of the CCM and Nurse Practitioners in Family Medicine

1. *Self-management support*: Provide methods and opportunities for patients to be empowered and prepared to manage their health conditions and health care. A self-management tool developed at the University of Michigan was adopted and a section added at the bottom of the tool to document the patient's hemoglobin A_{1C} (HbA_{1C}), blood pressure (BP), and low-density lipoprotein (LDL) cholesterol. This tool was used at every visit to document the patient's self-management goal. The patient chooses his or her goal, and the FNP and patient plan how they can best achieve it. Next the evidence-based targets for HbA_{1C}, BP, and LDL are reviewed and compared with the patient's results, and the plan to achieve the patient's goal values is documented. A copy of the plan is given to the patient and placed in the chart for the doctors and nurses to review at subsequent visits.
2. *Decision support*: Enhance and promote evidence-based clinical care that recognizes patient preferences. The diabetes care flow chart was updated to reflect current diabetes care guidelines. This chart is placed in front of the paper chart and serves as a summary for all providers to quickly review current values and

care given. Nursing staff were trained to update this flow chart at each visit, thus presenting patients with a proactive prepared summary for the provider to review before patient interaction. It definitely takes teamwork to keep a patient with diabetes care current, as even the best physician may not remember to ask about annual care requirements, such as annual ophthalmology examinations at each visit. The FNP and Registered Dietician are both certified diabetes educators with more than 40 years of diabetes clinical experience combined. The team serves as a resource for practical strategies in medication adjustment that are not all made explicit in practice guidelines.

3. *Delivery system design*: Promote proactive delivery of clinical care and support self-management within the system. The medical assistants and licensed vocational nurses are trained to ask the patient about their self-management goals as they room them, check on the last visit to the ophthalmologist, and prepare the patient for a lower extremity amputation prevention (LEAP) monofilament bilateral foot examination. The back-office staff has access to the Web-based Pay for Performance (P4P) registry, and uses this to note lapses in all measures of preventative care. This assists the entire team in ensuring that important process measures are completed for key age-appropriate preventive measures.

4. *Community resources and policies*: Identify and mobilize community-based resources to help meet the health care management needs of patients. The most important immediate aspect of a patient's community is the personal support system. The providers routinely assess a patent's support system, and encourage patients to bring a family member to every visit. Family members are instrumental in either supporting or undermining a patient's self-management efforts. The team help explain the difference between what a patient may perceive as nagging as opposed to gentle encouragement from family members. The author's new patient education packet was chosen specifically because the last page lists trusted national sources of patient education support. This tool also has phone numbers for patients without computer access or savvy. This publication, called *4 Steps to Control Your Diabetes. For Life*, is available from The US Department of Health and Human Services National Diabetes Education Program.

5. *Organizational support*: Leadership at all levels provides mechanisms to enhance care and improvements. The Department of Family Medicine has been extremely supportive of the FNP by recognizing the unique skills a nurse practitioner brings to the chronic disease management team. In the beginning, support was provided for a team to attend the California Chronic Care Coalition (CCCC), which allowed the FNP to focus on patient care and staff education while others helped to maintain the registry of patients with diabetes, monitor team efforts, and write reports. For the past year the University of California, Los Angeles has invested considerable time, money, and energy in primary care redesign to reflect the principles of the PCMH. Patients and providers have benefited from the addition of a clinical pharmacist to see patients with diabetes as part of the redesign effort. The University has included the FNP as part of the practice redesign team that meets twice monthly.

6. *Clinical information systems*: Organize and use data to provide efficient and effective care. In the past the author's practice had a database for the P4P system that included about 70% of those patients with diabetes. On request, a diabetes database for all payers has now been made available. There are 2 additional databases in place. The first is a list of all patients identified at the health plan level as having a family health center physician with key demographics and individual patient Hierarchal Category Codes (HCC) and Risk Adjustment Factor (RAF) scores. This list

allows us the team to quickly find the most ill patients as well as identify patients overutilizing the emergency department and having frequent hospital admissions, the so-called hot-spotters. This database was developed for 5 practices, as part of the primary care redesign/PCMH initiative. The university plans to rapidly expand this useful database to several additional practices by 2013. The second database identifies in real time hospital admission and discharges, and the same for the emergency room for both of the health system hospitals. Initially this information was sent via Fax for only 1 of the 2 hospitals. Now, both the inpatient and emergency-room patient use are received via email daily, with a summary provided monthly. The nurse practitioner helped to create the data included in the monthly summary.

FOCUS ON PRACTICE QUALITY AND SAFETY
Daily Reports Reviewed

The FNP reviews ancillary reports including laboratory, pathology, radiology, and other reports on abnormal results on a daily basis to all providers. In addition to trending abnormal results, the FNP reviews individual patients' appointment history, and assists in coordinating past and future care to ensure continuity. In addition to providing a smooth hand-off to the ordering provider, this activity also provides a safety net if the ordering provider is out of the office, where the FNP assists by contacting the patient and providing clinically appropriate follow-up instructions. This activity takes from 1 to 2 hours each day, depending on the number of reports. The benefit of this system ensures that 2 individuals, trained to back up each other thereby avoiding errors that can occur in a large practice with multiple providers, review ancillary reports. Moving forward, assigning a full-time care coordinator to assist the FNP in care coordination is anticipated.

Abnormal Electrocardiogram Reports

All abnormal electrocardiogram (ECG) reports are reviewed on a daily basis. The FNP receives the abnormal ECG reports and reviews the patient's paper record to determine if there is documentation that the ECG was ordered, if the reading from cardiology matches the family physician's impression. In addition, the physician's plan of care for an abnormal ECG is reviewed to ensure that the patient has clinically appropriate follow-up. We can all easily agree that in a busy practice, an abnormal ECG should not be placed in an in-basket or mailbox without knowledge of when the ordering doctor may address it.

Abnormal Pap Smears

How do you make sure that all women with an abnormal Papanicolaou smear (pap) receive the appropriate follow-up care? Do you have a running log and someone to coordinate their care? And can you hand this off to someone who can explain the treatment, sequelae, and implications for future childbearing in an articulate, caring manner that is appropriate to the patient's educational and developmental level? The FNP's role in addressing these important quality and safety issues involves maintaining an abnormal pap log, updated daily and reviewed monthly. Patients who have not received care are scheduled for follow-up, and if the patient is unable to be contacted then a certified letter is sent to the patient requesting they contact the FNP. Because this database has been maintained for more than 8 years, the practice is able to benchmark trends in the number of abnormal results including unsatisfactory results.

Anticoagulation Clinic

Within the author's university health system there exists a sophisticated anticoagulation clinic where the majority of patients on warfarin are monitored. The health system clinic is located on the main campus in a busy area with significant parking fees. Patients prefer to come to their family health center where they receive their primary care and where there currently is free parking. The FNP does not initiate warfarin but makes adjustments to ensure time in the international normalized ratio (INR) range is within an acceptable benchmark. At any given time, the FNP manages approximately 50 patients. During their visit with the FNP, the patients have acute and chronic issues addressed as well as on-site INR results and adjustments to their dose in real time. Faculty and resident physicians refer patients to the FNP anticoagulation clinic. The FNP maintains a database with INR results and reports the percentage of INR values in range on a monthly basis.

Medication Refill Requests and Prior Authorizations

All primary care practices receive medication refill requests on a daily basis, and in the author's practice the FNP receives 20 to 60 requests for medication refills per day in a practice with 35,000 annual patient visits. There is a handful of faculty physicians in the practice who choose to review and respond to patient refill requests. Studies of prescribing patterns within the practice indicate that the number of refill requests a physician receives is influenced by how they practice and communicate with their patients. At this clinic, for the majority of prescription refills, there is a centralized system for medication refill requests that uses the FNP.

Using electronic prescribing software, all medication refill requests are entered into the e-prescribing system. The medical record staff compiles the medical records, faxes, and phone requests for refills throughout the day. Information for each medication request includes the last visit, next visit, and the patient's primary care physician. The FNP reviews the medical record and reconciles the medication request with the last medication dose and directions documented in the clinic record. After review and clarification with the patient and/or prescriber, the prescription is e-prescribed. In addition, during the process care coordination for preventive care is also reviewed. An email listing patients who need to be followed up for medication management and preventive care is sent to staff members whose task it is to call patients and schedule follow-up visits. Although this activity ranges from 1 to 3 hours, the added value of a nurse practitioner performing medication review and care coordination as well as an experienced set of clinical eyes reviewing family medicine resident care has averted duplicate and wrong-dose errors.

Recently, the FNP took over the prior authorization process that had proved to be a time-consuming process for a registered nurse. With systems and process expertise as well as the ability to prescribe medications without requiring a doctor's signature to change medications, the prior authorization process has significantly been improved by using the FNP.

POPULATION MANAGEMENT FOR QUALITY
Pay for Performance

For the past 8 years the author's practice has worked to manage the P4P patient population. Over the years, the report has evolved and is updated monthly, and identifies for all patients their unique medical record number, demographic data, performance-measure laboratory data, last appointment where a service related to the condition being monitored occurred, and the last visit within the health system. The practice has tried various methods to contact patients who are either missing care or who need care coordination/intensification. From chart checks to phone calls, the FNP has been very instrumental in assisting the team in improving performance and ultimately the care of patients.

Insurance Carrier Reports/Requests

Physicians receive a weekly flood of requests for patient information from insurance carriers. Similar to P4P, these companies are asking for patient updates or noting gaps in care. The FNP receives these reports for the entire practice, and either sends documentation of care requested or calls the patient to coordinate care. The FNP also handles all requests for HEDIS (Healthcare Effectiveness Data and Information Set) measures from the copious number of different insurance carriers. A full-time care coordinator will be hired as part of practice redesign to provide assistance to the FNP, thus allowing her to practice to the top of her license.

Compliance and Regulatory Audits

The FNP was called on to merge 2 practices, and provided leadership in the role of nursing supervisor for a period of 3 years. During this time the FNP learned about the compliance and regulatory aspects of a family medicine practice. She trained the staff to be "audit ready every day" rather than ramping up for audits. In addition to the billing and coding audits for which she participates, facility site review and program-specific audits occur every 2 years. These audits include the Vaccine for Children Program to ensure the practice is compliant and current with evidence-based immunization practices; the Children with Disabilities Program audit aimed to provide preventive well-child care; and Medicaid HMO audits for some of the sickest and most vulnerable patients. Given that the FNP is able to assess clinical care, she is able to quickly note gaps in clinical care and develop plans to remedy these problems effectively and efficiently.

TRAVEL MEDICINE

Pretravel care is primary prevention and falls easily within the skill set of an FNP. The FNP in the author's practice has been providing travel advice, vaccines, and prophylaxis against malaria and other illnesses for 10 years. It has been found that requesting payments for travel vaccines at the time of the visit is best practice.

MOTIVATIONAL INTERVIEWING

FNPs view patients holistically, involve family members, and educate and motivate patients. FNPs use motivational interviewing at every visit and according to Harris and colleagues,[9] this type of interview acknowledges that:

Most people move through a series of steps to change their behavior
Effective change is self-directed
Confrontation and negative messages are ineffective
Knowledge does not equal behavior change
Reducing ambivalence is the key to change

This type of interaction is less of a lecture and more of a discussion or a negotiation. As nurses, we acknowledge that each patient is an individual with his or her own set of beliefs, culture, life experiences, and psychological strengths/weaknesses. Motivational interviewing takes practice and time to be effective. For many chronic diseases, making the diagnosis and directing the treatment is straightforward, whereas helping patients to adopt lifestyle changes necessary for self-management of their chronic disease is quite challenging. Most doctors would appreciate having an educated professional to whom they could refer their patients for the type of interaction that will make their treatments more effective. Nurse practitioners are a valuable resource for chronic disease.

HOW TO HIRE A NURSE PRACTITIONER

1. Advertise the position on-line, in journals, and through state and national nurse practitioner organizations.
2. Understand nurse practitioner education. Look for a nurse practitioner with both a Baccalaureate and Master's degree in nursing.
3. Understand nurse practitioner certification. There are 2 main groups who offer certification: The American Nurses Credentialing Center and the American Academy of Nurse Practitioners. These groups provide entry-level competency-based examinations reflective of nurse practitioner knowledge and expertise.
4. Know your state laws. Every state has different laws that regulate nurse practitioner practice. You can contact your state's Board of Registered Nursing for current nurse practitioner practice laws. Nurse practitioners in California practice under standardized protocols. These documents, outlining which functions nurse practitioners are allowed to perform independently, have been developed and signed by supervising physicians.
5. Understand prescription privileges. All 50 states allow nurse practitioners to write prescriptions. Only Florida and Alabama do not allow nurse practitioners to write for controlled substances. States vary on how prescriptions are to be written. In California, one "furnishes" and does not "prescribe." Nurse practitioners are required to demonstrate pharmaceutical knowledge by passing an approved course and having 1500 physician-supervised prescribing hours when applying for a furnishing number. The name of the supervising physician must be on the prescription and there must be a formulary, written as a standardized procedure, which outlines the medications nurse practitioners are able to furnish independently.
6. Interview for experience. There were an estimated 9500 new nurse practitioners completing academic programs in 2010-2011. A new nurse practitioner needs at least 6 months to a year of working closely with a physician or experienced nurse practitioner to gain the diagnostic and treatment skills needed to begin to practice independently. Of course a more experienced nurse practitioner can function independently quite rapidly.
7. Understand billing. Both Medicare and Medicaid programs allow for nurse practitioners to bill independently but reimburse at 85% of physician charges. If a nurse practitioner bills "incident to," then care may be billed under the supervising physician who must also cosign the progress note. Incident to billing reimburses at 100% of the physician rate.

SUMMARY

As advanced practice nurses, nurse practitioners have a unique skill set. Their basic nursing knowledge provides the foundation for patient-centered care. The additional diagnosis and treatment skills create competency in health maintenance, acute care, and chronic disease management. Nurse practitioners are capable leaders in primary care design as practices nationwide move to consider and adopt the PCMH. The CCM provides a structure to enhance the care of chronic illness. Nurse practitioners are instrumental in many areas of this model as both leaders and caregivers. Safety and quality are basic medical home goals; nurse practitioners enhance both. If you are striving to provide the very best for your patients, consider adding a nurse practitioner to your practice. You will find this to be an effective "value add" in every way.

REFERENCES

1. Available at: http://www.aanp.org/all-about-nps/np-fact-sheet. Accessed June, 2012.
2. Available at: http://www.aanp.org/all-about-nps/what-is-an-np. Accessed June, 2012.
3. Available at: http://www.ncqa.org/tabid/631/Default.aspx. Definition Patient Centered Medical Home. Accessed July, 2012.
4. Available at: http://www.aafp.org/online/en/home/media/releases/2012/transformed-memorial-hermann.html.
5. California Academic Chronic Care Collaborative (CA ACCC). Available at: http://www.chcf.org/projects/2010/california-academic-chronic-care-collaborative#ixzz23 NOgcfYY.
6. Available at: http://www.improvingchroniccare.org/index.php?p=Model_Elements &s=18. 2003.
7. Available at: http://www.improvingchroniccare.org/index.php?p=Model_Elements &s=18. Six elements of the chronic care model.
8. Available at: http://ndep.nih.gov/publications. 4 Steps to Control Your Diabetes. For Life.
9. Harris R, Aldea M, Kirkley D. A motivational interviewing and common factors approach to change in working with alcohol use and abuse in college students. Prof Psychol Res Pract 2006;37(6):614–21.

Integration of Behavioral Medicine in Primary Care

Michelle Anne Bholat, MD, MPH*, Lara Ray, PhD,
Matthew Brensilver, PhD, Kimberly Ling, PhD, Steven Shoptaw, PhD

KEYWORDS

• Behavioral medicine • Primary care • Integration • Organization

KEY POINTS

- Incorporating behavioral medicine in the delivery of care offers a wide range of opportunities to implement sustainable changes in the health care system.
- Within primary care settings, pain disorders, addiction, depression, and anxiety disorders are highly prevalent. In addition, numerous chronic health conditions require behavioral support for lifestyle change. These disorders are optimally managed through interdisciplinary collaborations that include a behavioral medicine component.
- Extant models of behavioral medicine in primary care settings have lacked the qualities of truly integrative, interdisciplinary collaborations.

The current health care system is broken and there are many incentives to identify ways to implement and to sustain changes for physicians, for clinics and hospitals, for patients, and for payers. Employers and employees are paying more for health care coverage than ever and are getting fewer covered services. Co-pays and annual deductibles are high, leading many patients to postpone or to default on preventive and routine health care. Primary care patients increasingly display high levels of complexity in terms of both medical and psychological conditions. In California, the breadth of services offered by primary care physicians has also increased, whereas payments for those services have stayed the same or decreased. Patients who are uninsured and who use emergency department services for problems most efficiently treated in primary care settings default on huge bills, creating costs that ultimately are passed on to patients with health coverage in the form of continually rising costs for health care. These changes are happening while primary care clinics increasingly manage patients with chronic diseases.[1]

This challenging, but chronic, condition of the health care landscape calls for interdisciplinary and integrative approaches that promote delivery of efficient,

The authors gratefully acknowledge NIH training grant T32DA 024600 on Addiction Medicine in Primary Care (Shoptaw PI).
UCLA Family Health Center, 1920 Colorado Avenue, Santa Monica, CA 90404, USA
* Corresponding author.
E-mail address: mbholat@mednet.ucla.edu

Prim Care Clin Office Pract 39 (2012) 605–614
http://dx.doi.org/10.1016/j.pop.2012.08.003   **primarycare.theclinics.com**
0095-4543/12/$ – see front matter © 2012 Published by Elsevier Inc.

cost-effective, and high-quality medical care. No medication can cure chronic diseases. Instead, behavior change is required to manage the impacts of chronic diseases on an ongoing basis. Integration of behavioral medicine and primary care represents an alternative to delivering comprehensive, high-quality care to patients, and, in doing so, forges new relationships within the health care team and administrative leadership. However, few models exist to guide the integration of this team-based approach into primary care settings, in which the predominant model consists of care being delivered by the individual provider. This article reviews the rationale for undertaking the integration of behavioral medicine in primary care and describes the experience of the UCLA Family Health Center in integrating behavioral medicine into an urban, primary care, patient-centered medical home that provides services to a mix of insured and underinsured patients.

RATIONALE

As patients increasingly present to primary care with chronic conditions, they require more than prescriptions from their doctors to teach and maintain positive health outcomes. Given time constraints, these needs are best addressed by an interdisciplinary team that has an explicit focus on prescribing medications in the context of sustained behavior change.[2,3] The team can extend the physician by focusing on behavioral domains that range from medication adherence to lifestyle factors (dietary changes, exercise) to behavioral care approaches for mental health, addiction, and pain disorders that are both highly prevalent and comorbid with other chronic illnesses.

Showing that primary care can breach the gap, general medical care settings now represent an important sector for the treatment of mental health disorders. For example, care for depression in general medical practice more than doubled in a comparison of data from 1990 to 1992 and 2001 to 2003.[4,5] Further, exclusive reliance on general medical providers without support from a psychiatrist or mental health specialist increased by 153% during the same period.[6,7] A similar pattern may be developing regarding the treatment of addictions, with the recent approval of a palette of medications. As with mental illness, substance abuse disorders are highly prevalent. An estimated 22.1 million Americans have substance abuse or dependence, excepting tobacco dependence,[8] with more than two-thirds of these visiting primary care doctors regularly.[9] The increased access to mental health services in primary care coupled with the decreased stigma of seeking treatment of a substance disorder and/or mental illness in these settings is critical to reaching individuals affected by these illnesses. This point is particularly relevant because the consequences of addictions and mental illness are disproportionate for those living with economic and health care disparities.

The primary care setting also allows for a developmental lifespan approach to identifying and treating mild-to-moderate mental health and addiction disorders. Adolescents and young adults are more likely to use substances than all other age groups,[10] with the incidence of drug abuse and dependence disorders peaking at ages 19 to 25 years.[11] This pattern coincides with initial onset of major mental illnesses. To that end, primary care clinicians are in a unique position to serve sentinel and early intervention functions. Across the lifespan, alcohol and drug problems can emerge when patients use these substances to cope with family problems, chronic pain, and economic hardships, which are situations that also are detectable by primary care physicians. Concerns about substance use no longer remit with advanced age, because older adults (baby boomers) are now aging up, but not out, of substance use, particularly marijuana. Again, the primary care clinic represents an ideal setting for identifying and treating mild-to-moderate metal health problems, including substance misuse.

Several physical and organizational factors serve to maintain separate silos for primary medical care, substance abuse treatment, and mental health care. There is no systematic approach to providing behavioral health in primary care settings and, without 1 or more behavioral health specialists and physician champions to advocate change, the inertia of the status quo often prevails. Concerns over billing and reimbursement for behavioral health services predominate because primary care clinics operate on tight margins that preclude providing services that are not (at least) budget neutral. Physicians typically avoid discussions about addiction with their patients, believing there may not be much they can do to help, which may reflect stigma and inadequate training.[12] A notable exception is the increasing willingness of physicians to discuss tobacco smoking and cessation.

EPIDEMIOLOGY

The need for integrating behavioral health into primary care is great. The prevalence of mental health or addiction disorders in primary care is high and increases substantially when factoring in mental health, addiction, or pain disorders that are comorbid to chronic diseases. This article reviews the prevalence of these disorders with a focus on primary care settings.

Depression and Anxiety

Depression and anxiety disorders are common in primary care. In a large representative sample of US adults, 26.2% had at least 1 past-year mental disorder, with anxiety (18.1%) and mood disorders (9.5%) figuring most prominently.[4] In primary care practices, depression or dysthymia diagnoses were observed in 27% to 29% of patients; anxiety disorders were observed in 19% to 26% of patients.[13–15] These figures are striking given that only 5% of patients visited their provider for a psychiatric complaint and that most patients with current depressive disorders do not receive mental health treatment. Depression also is commonly comorbid to diabetes mellitus,[16] to coronary artery disease,[17] and to stroke.[18] Untreated depression is associated with difficulties in accessing primary care and obtaining comprehensive services; 2 critical markers of quality of care.[19] To that end, the cost of care for depressed older adults is significantly increased for both ambulatory and inpatient services.[20] It is commonly accepted that depression is a distinguishing feature of high users of medical services.[21]

Addiction

About 1 in 11 American adults older than 12 years met criteria for substance abuse or dependence[8]; alcohol abuse and dependence represent most cases (17.9 million; 7.0% of adults and 81% of the total substance abuse/dependence population). Heavy alcohol use is associated with a huge public health burden[22] and most (70%–80%) individuals with problematic drinking and drug abuse do not seek treatment.[23] Primary care clinics have been identified as an important resource in using Screening, Brief Interventions, Referral to Treatment (SBIRT) procedures to identify and to make appropriate dispositions of cases based on levels of use or nonuse.[23] A growing number of medications for addictive disorders, whose efficacy is boosted by providing short-term behavioral therapies, are available for use in outpatient settings (**Table 1**). In addition to identifying patients with addiction problems in primary care settings, intervention with mild-to-moderate cases may reduce stigma and circumvent barriers to treatments in individuals who would be unlikely to seek care at a specialty clinic.

Table 1
Evidence-based medication and behavioral treatments for substance use disorders

Medications Approved for Use	
Smoking	Nicotine replacement therapy, bupropion, varenicline
Opioids	Methadone, buprenorphine, naltrexone
Alcohol	Oral and injectable naltrexone, acamprosate, disulfiram
Methamphetamine	Strong signal for bupropion
Behavioral Therapy Models with Efficacy	
Cognitive behavior therapy	Smoking, opioids, alcohol, stimulant disorders
Contingency management	Stimulant disorders
Motivational interviewing	Smoking, alcohol, stimulant disorders
12-step facilitation	Alcohol disorders

Pain

Chronic noncancer pain (typically defined as pain persisting longer than 3 months) affects a large proportion of the population. Prevalence is estimated to be approximately 20%,[24,25] although representative surveys find rates exceeding 30%.[26,27] As the prevalence and burden of chronic pain has been more fully recognized, the last 2 decades have seen large increases in opioid prescribing rates,[28] resulting in an estimated 10 million Americans currently receiving chronic opioid treatment. Those at increased risk for prescribed opioid misuse include individuals with comorbid psychiatric disorders,[29] younger individuals, and those with prior substance abuse problems.[30] Annual direct medical expenditure is in the tens of billions of dollars,[31] with associated losses in economic productivity estimated in excess of $60 billion.[32] For low back pain, for example, primary care costs represent 13% of direct medical expenditures, comparable with inpatient services (17%) and pharmacy (13%).[33] Behavioral interventions targeting functional impairment and depressive symptoms associated with chronic pain have been advanced as means of addressing this public health burden.[34] These figures highlight the potential value of behavioral medicine in mitigating some of the consequences and health impacts that lie at the intersection of chronic pain, opioid treatment, and substance misuse or addiction.

INTEGRATION OF BEHAVIORAL MEDICINE INTO PRIMARY CARE: PREPARATIONS

Moving from a primary care clinic to a patient-centered medical home with an integrated model that includes behavioral medicine as an essential part of the clinic takes time, foresight, and patience. In the early phase, introducing behavioral medicine, with its focus on mitigating impacts of chronic diseases, into an urban primary care clinic requires administrative and clinical leadership to be not only a champion, but a booster. With time, goodwill will be forthcoming from nursing staff and other clinicians who observe positive outcomes for patients who access behavioral medicine services. However, foresight is vital. Executive leadership's prospective definition of the level of integration for the behavioral medicine clinic in primary care ranges from minimal (refer patients in primary care to specialty clinics) to basic (having behavioral health providers close by or on-site) to close (behavioral health is partially or fully integrated). Fully integrated behavioral health in primary care contains (1) screening for comorbid conditions, (2) embedded behavioral health staff, (3) active linking of patients to services, (4) roaming consultants or accessible telemedicine services that can aid cases that emerge during clinic, and (5) continuity of care (ie, returning the patient to the primary care provider). Full integration requires support from leadership during the introduction of the services, while also retaining perspective over the long term as the system accommodates to service provision and begins to experience its benefits and unique challenges.

At all stages, from introduction to consolidation to maintenance, a fully integrated model of behavioral health in primary care requires formalized regular communication, care coordination, and case management between primary care physicians, the behavioral specialist, and the support of the health care team, which includes both front and back office staff members. Problems that arise when integrating behavioral health into primary care often signal inadequate, unclear, or insufficient levels of communication between physicians, nurses/back office staff, behavioral specialists, and administrative support staff. One mechanism for communicating in multidisciplinary or team practice settings is a huddle, or a period before clinic when all members of the team meet briefly to share information about patients on the schedule to prepare the team for cases that may need extra attention or support. Communication using a brief consult or an e-mail regarding the diagnosis and expected treatment plan for a patient aids case coordination and team building. Preparation of a discharge summary by the behavioral medicine team, which is complete with concrete behavioral recommendations that can help the primary care physician evaluate and support healthy behavior change, is essential.

Developing methods for frequent formal and informal communication between team members facilitates smoother operations when integrating behavioral medicine into primary care. Adequate forethought must be given to the documentation of behavioral health services in relation to the patient's medical record. Additional privacy issues require consideration when documenting care, particularly in cases in which mental health and substance abuse diagnoses are involved, because these invoke higher levels of requirements for privacy and restrictions on who can access progress notes or other documentation. Privacy issues are particularly important in clinic settings that have already migrated from paper charts to electronic health records. A separation of behavioral medicine records from medical records may be recommended to meet the requirements for confidentiality associated with mental health records. It is important that the organization addresses how key information such as a complete medication list that includes psychiatric and addiction medications, as well as access to behavioral health records by need-to-know medical staff, must be adequately addressed by executive leadership to ensure safe and effective medical care to the patient.

At the start and periodically afterward, consideration of clinic forms and patient registries with outcome measures and metrics for assessing progress is essential. Documents for legal and billing purposes likely exist and require minor alterations, including consent/assent documents, releases of information, agreements regarding billing, charge documents, treatment plans, progress notes, and discharge summaries. Further, valid and reliable behavioral medicine domain measurements are available. These measures include domains of somatic complaints, depression and anxiety symptoms, functional impairment, and quality of life. Behavioral markers likely have the most profound strength in showing changes that correspond with provision of behavioral medicine services. These markers include number of visits to high-intensity medical care settings before and after behavioral medicine services are delivered (eg, emergency departments, hospital), percent arrival to scheduled primary care appointments before and following behavioral medicine services, and number of sessions attended during behavioral medicine treatment. Settings that have access to electronic medical records can more easily gather some of these metrics, whereas others may require the addition of paper-and-pencil (or computerized) instruments.

A UNIFIED BEHAVIORAL MEDICINE SERVICE: CASE EXAMPLE

In January 2009, our team integrated behavioral medicine into the UCLA Family Health Center (UFHC). In the behavioral medicine clinic, patients receive care from a multidisciplinary team that may include their referring family physician, an addiction medicine specialist, a pain management specialist (if required), and a behavioral medicine specialist, which results in coordination of primary care, pharmacotherapy (for medical, psychological, and pain conditions), brief (5–8 weeks) behavioral treatment, and assessment and treatment (or referral) for substance abuse in 1 facility. Communication is facilitated by a huddle before the weekly behavioral medicine clinic to coordinate concerns regarding shared patients with front and back office staff, physician, and clinic managers and creates integrated treatment plans to best support the patient. In between the clinic visits, the patient-centered medical home team meets via teleconference every other week for 60 minutes to review cases that require further discussion and as frequently as needed to address urgent issues.

All treatments delivered by the behavioral medicine clinic are short term, averaging 5 to 8 sessions, and are delivered using evidence-based models. Although evidence-based models are used, flexibility (ie, practical counseling) guides the delivery of these interventions. This flexibility is essential given the complex clinical presentations that are typical. A unitary, focused approach dictated by a single treatment manual generally fails to address the diverse needs of patients seen in our clinic. For example, behavior treatment manuals often fail to account for medication compliance and other medical health indices that are crucial to the primary care setting. In addition to the interplay of chronic diseases many of our patients present with, more than a single psychiatric diagnosis is common, a pattern found in nationally representative samples.[35] There is a dearth of evidence to guide decisions regarding adaptation of evidence-based psychosocial treatments to complex cases, leaving the clinician tasked with tailoring the intervention[36] to the client's presentation. The clinician may select a specific evidence-based intervention for the presenting concern, but elements of other empirically validated treatment models are often grafted onto the primary intervention. For example, case management is usually required to coordinate care and to avoid duplication between providers. As patients complete a course of treatment with the behavioral medicine clinic, the referring physician is routinely provided with recommendations for ongoing management to sustain, and perhaps enhance, gains. All behavioral medicine services are provided under the direct supervision of licensed clinical psychologists. Consistent with an attending model of care, the attending clinical psychologists join the master's-level clinicians for a portion of each visit, to ensure that the treatment goals were appropriately identified and that the recommended interventions were implemented flexibly and effectively.

Treatment is brief, with the initial contract typically being 5 sessions following the initial assessment. As signaled earlier, the primary objective for the patient is improved functioning (ie, avoiding emergency medical care, ability to return to work); improvements in mood and affect are desirable, but are secondary. This focus helps clinicians to avoid drift in treatment and to focus on relieving impairments from presenting symptoms. Although features of personality disorders are prominent in many of our patients, we do not directly challenge these traits and instead seek progress on the presenting complaints and reinforce patients' progress toward health. Where appropriate, patients who may benefit are referred for longer-term care. Preliminary qualitative data from initial patients treated show that session attendance corresponds with improvements in overall clinical ratings such that those who were rated as mildly to moderately improved averaged 6 to 8 sessions, whereas those who were rated as showing no improvement or continued deterioration of functioning averaged 2 or fewer sessions.

Successful implementation of a behavioral medicine clinic within an urban family medicine teaching/innovation center in a university medical department required coordination of individual, group, and organizational interests. In 2005, the academic roles of addiction and behavioral medicine expertise were integrated into the Family Medicine department. In 2006, the team conducted a clinical trial within the primary care clinic, integrating the academic research group with the primary care clinic team. In 2008, additional institutional support was gained by colocating addiction medicine, behavioral medicine, pain, and palliative care in the Family Medicine department. In 2009, the behavioral and addiction medicine services were offered to patients. In addition, a National Institute of Health training grant for fellows and post-doctoral trainees as well as a practicum for advanced clinical psychology graduate students were established, providing training opportunities and foundations for research. As the clinic developed, standardized procedures were developed to assist the coordination and integration of the primary care and behavioral medicine. Innovations were introduced and tested using Rapid Cycle Improvement Plan-Do-Study-Act methodology to implement changes quickly, receive feedback, and revise procedures. Standardized charts and measures were used to reduce redundancies and increase consistency in information. Brief meetings or huddles were instituted at the beginning of each clinic day to quickly review up-to-the-minute patient needs, including ensuring coordination when patients were seeing multiple care providers, confirming that new patients were provided with the appropriate previsit materials and introduced to all members of the team, and making certain that patients discharged from the behavioral care team were receiving appropriate and timely access to follow-up care. One additional marker of success was that the behavioral medicine reached financial viability in 2010, 1 year after implementation.

LESSONS LEARNED

At this point, behavioral medicine is a cost-effective addition to an urban and university-based family medicine practice. In addition to being well-received by patients and clinicians alike, there are multiple signs that integration of behavioral medicine has impacted the clinic: (1) staff members recognize that (for the most part) patients enrolled in behavioral medicine get better, as marked by reductions in no-shows/cancellations; (2) team treatment concepts are spreading, and the huddle initially linked to behavioral medicine is now used with additional team members within the clinic; (3) increased and focused communication about behavioral science and the ways it can be used by all members of the team has reduced the overall number of episodes with difficult patients requiring attention from the medical staff or police. Although the behavioral medicine clinic is a work in progress, there are more successes than failures at the level of the patients, of the clinical team, and of the bottom line.

This example of integrating behavioral medicine into primary care at UCLA may not generalize to all primary care settings. The assemblage of champions in administration, skilled behavioral specialists, and supportive team members willing to work toward financial viability may be uncommon. In those clinics where champions in administration, skilled behavioral specialists, and supportive team members are colocated, front office staff and other providers and administrators may require time to adjust to care delivery that deviates from the individual provider model. In addition, it is necessary to refresh the soul. There are multiple successes along the way that show the important ways that the lives of patients who receive behavioral medicine can be profoundly changed (see the case example).

CASE EXAMPLE: GERARDO

Gerardo is a middle-aged Hispanic man with paranoid schizophrenia and alcohol dependence who lives alone in a low-cost care facility. He was referred to behavioral medicine services because of required emergency department treatment following drinking binges every 3 to 4 months. Gerardo was referred to behavioral medicine after it was determined that high liver function tests prevented use of naltrexone for alcohol dependence.

At intake, Gerardo and his clinician agreed to work toward alcohol abstinence using contingency management (ie, an evidence-based treatment that provides financial rewards in exchange for biologic or other observed markers of substance abstinence). This decision was made after noting that Gerardo enjoyed attending Alcoholics Anonymous (AA) meetings; it gave him something to do and he enjoyed the stories. However, his suspiciousness interfered with him becoming actively involved with the social aspects of the program. Gerardo did not drink on days when he attended the AA meetings.

Because there is no inexpensive biomarker of binge drinking, we designed a contingency management schedule that provided Gerardo with a $5 coupon for a local fast food restaurant in exchange for a signature card documenting attendance at AA meetings on 6 of 7 days per week. Gerardo was able to meet this criterion quickly and within a few weeks was regularly attending meetings daily. He stopped binge drinking. He delighted in the reinforcement when he exchanged his signed attendance logs for a $5 gift coupon. The behavioral specialist noted that Gerardo's ability to avoid binge drinking was stable. In a later session, the topic of appearance and hygiene was discussed. The next session Gerardo attended clinic freshly shaved, with a new haircut and clean clothes.

After about 3 months, we provided a report to the referring primary care physician describing how to continue the contingency management schedule, with recommendations of fading the reinforcements as sustained abstinence continued. Gerardo continues to maintain abstinence. His physician is discussing potential treatment with depot naltrexone as a prophylactic to binge drinking given that he no longer receives contingency management.

REFERENCES

1. Bodenheimer T, Chen E, Bennett HD. Confronting the growing burden of chronic disease: can the U. S. health care workforce do the job? Health Aff 2009;28(1): 64–74.
2. Croghan TW, Brown JD. Integrating mental health treatment into the patient centered medical home. (Prepared by Mathematica Policy Research under Contract No. HHSA290200900019I TO2.) AHRQ Publication No. 10-0084-EF. Rockville (MD): Agency for Healthcare Research and Quality; 2010.
3. Pruitt SD, Klapow JC, Epping-Jordan JA, et al. Moving behavioral medicine to the front line: a model for the integration of behavioral and medical sciences in primary care. Prof Psychol Res Pr 1998;29(3):230.
4. Kessler RC, Chiu WT, Demler O, et al. Prevalence, severity, and comorbidity of 12-month DSM-IV disorders in the National Comorbidity Survey Replication. Arch Gen Psychiatry 2005;62(6):617.

5. Kessler RC, Demler O, Frank RG, et al. Prevalence and treatment of mental disorders, 1990 to 2003. N Engl J Med 2005;352(24):2515–23.
6. Wang PS, Demler O, Olfson M, et al. Changing profiles of service sectors used for mental health care in the US. Am J Psychiatry 2006;163(7):1187.
7. Westen D, Novotny CM, Thompson-Brenner H. The empirical status of empirically supported psychotherapies: assumptions, findings, and reporting in controlled clinical trials. Psychol Bull 2004;130(4):631.
8. National Survey on Drug Use and Health. 2011.
9. Whitlock, et al. 2002.
10. SAMHSA. 2007.
11. Compton, et al. 2007.
12. Soyka M, Gorelick DA. Why should addiction medicine be an attractive field for young physicians? Addiction 2009;104(2):169–72.
13. Ansseau M, Dierick M, Buntinkx F, et al. High prevalence of mental disorders in primary care. J Affect Disord 2004;78(1):49–55.
14. Kroenke K, Spitzer RL, Williams JB, et al. Anxiety disorders in primary care: prevalence, impairment, comorbidity, and detection. Ann Intern Med 2007;146(5): 317–25.
15. Roca M, Gili M, Garcia-Garcia M, et al. Prevalence and comorbidity of common mental disorders in primary care. J Affect Disord 2009;119(1–3):52–8.
16. Anderson, Freedland, Clouse, et al. 2001.
17. Musselman DL, Evans DL, Nemeroff CB. The relationship of depression to cardiovascular disease: epidemiology, biology, and treatment. Arch Gen Psychiatry 1998;55(7):580.
18. Burvill P, Johnson G, Jamrozik K, et al. Prevalence of depression after stroke: the Perth Community Stroke Study. Br J Psychiatry 1995;166(3):320–7.
19. Druss BG, Rask K, Katon WJ. Major depression, depression treatment and quality of primary medical care. Gen Hosp Psychiatry 2008;30(1):20–5.
20. Katon WJ, Lin E, Russo J, et al. Increased medical costs of a population-based sample of depressed elderly patients. Arch Gen Psychiatry 2003;60(9):897.
21. Pearson SD, Katzelnick DJ, Simon GE, et al. Depression among high utilizers of medical care. J Gen Intern Med 1999;14(8):461–8.
22. Harwood H, Henrick D, Fountain D, et al. The economic costs of alcohol and drug abuse in the United States 1992. 2009.
23. Madras BK, Compton WM, Avula D, et al. Screening, brief interventions, referral to treatment (SBIRT) for illicit drug and alcohol use at multiple healthcare sites: comparison at intake and 6 months later. Drug Alcohol Depend 2009;99(1–3): 280–95.
24. Gureje O, Von Korff M, Simon GE, et al. Persistent pain and well-being. JAMA 1998;280(2):147–51.
25. Kerns RD, Sellinger J, Goodin BR. Psychological treatment of chronic pain. Annu Rev Clin Psychol 2011;7(1):411–34.
26. Johannes CB, Le TK, Zhou X, et al. The prevalence of chronic pain in United States adults: results of an internet-based survey. J Pain 2010;11(11):1230–9.
27. Munce SE, Stewart DE. Gender differences in depression and chronic pain conditions in a national epidemiologic survey. Psychosomatics 2007;48(5):394–9.
28. Okie S. A flood of opioids, a rising tide of deaths. N Engl J Med 2010;363(21): 1981–5.
29. Braden JB, Sullivan MD, Ray GT, et al. Trends in long-term opioid therapy for non-cancer pain among persons with a history of depression. Gen Hosp Psychiatry 2009;31(6):564–70.

30. Edlund MJ, Steffick D, Hudson T, et al. Risk factors for clinically recognized opioid abuse and dependence among veterans using opioids for chronic non-cancer pain. Pain 2007;129(3):355–62.
31. Luo X, Pietrobon R, Sun X, et al. Estimates and patterns of direct health care expenditures among individuals with back pain in the United States. Spine 2004;29(1):79–86.
32. Stewart WF, Ricci JA, Chee E, et al. Lost productive time and cost due to common pain conditions in the US workforce. JAMA 2003;290(18):2443–54.
33. Dagenais S, Caro J, Haldeman S. A systematic review of low back pain cost of illness studies in the United States and internationally. Spine J 2008;8(1):8–20.
34. Engel CC, Von Korff M, Katon WJ. Back pain in primary care: predictors of high health-care costs. Pain 1996;65(2):197–204.
35. Krueger RF, Markon KE. Reinterpreting comorbidity: a model-based approach to understanding and classifying psychopathology. Annu Rev Clin Psychol 2006;2: 111.
36. Ruscio AM, Holohan DR. Applying empirically supported treatments to complex cases: ethical, empirical, and practical considerations. Clin Psychol Sci Pract 2006;13(2):146–62.

Opportunities to Improve Clinical Outcomes and Challenges to Implementing Clinical Pharmacists into Health Care Teams

Alison Reta, PharmD[a],*, Anahita Dashtaei, PharmD[b],
Sokkim Lim, PharmD[c], Tina Nguyen, PharmD[d],
Michelle Anne Bholat, MD, MPH[a]

KEYWORDS

- Pharmacotherapy • Clinical pharmacists • Health care teams
- Clinical pharmacy services

KEY POINTS

- By addressing issues of medication non-adherence; evaluating proper dosing; ensuring correct administration; detecting potential for drug-food, drug-herb, drug-disease, and drug-drug interactions; and providing strategies to reduce adverse events, clinical pharmacists can potentially maximize the effectiveness of medications while consequently improving patient safety and clinical outcomes.
- With extensive knowledge of pharmacotherapy and the many facets of health care, clinical pharmacists are equipped with the skills necessary to improve outcomes for medical institutions and the patients they serve.
- More than 59% of drug-related emergency room visits are preventable[1] with the most common reasons including adverse drug reactions (39.3%), nonadherence (27.9%), and use of the wrong or suboptimal drug (11.5%).[2]

INTRODUCTION

In both inpatient and ambulatory care settings, clinical pharmacists incorporate their broad scope of pharmacotherapy knowledge with patient-specific factors to evaluate medication regimens. By addressing issues of medication nonadherence; evaluating proper dosing; ensuring correct administration; detecting potential for drug-food,

No disclosures reported.
[a] University of Southern California School of Pharmacy, Los Angeles, CA, USA; [b] Sharp Community Pharmacy, Coronado, CA, USA; [c] Cal eConnect, Inc, Emeryville, CA 94608, USA; [d] City of Hope National Medical Center, Duarte, CA, USA
* Corresponding author.
E-mail address: reta@usc.edu

Prim Care Clin Office Pract 39 (2012) 615–626
http://dx.doi.org/10.1016/j.pop.2012.08.005
0095-4543/12/$ – see front matter © 2012 Elsevier Inc. All rights reserved.

drug-herb, drug-disease and drug-drug interactions; and providing strategies to reduce adverse events, clinical pharmacists can potentially maximize the effectiveness of medications while consequently improving patient safety and clinical outcomes.

The overall training of pharmacists involves not only the mastery of pharmacologic knowledge but also legal, social, ethical, cultural, and economic principles that are essential in the provision of patient care. Clinical pharmacists undergo a rigorous 4-year didactic education through the pharmacy doctoral degree program, which includes coursework ranging from pharmacology and clinical therapeutics to health economics and management principles.[3] They build on this academic foundation through postgraduate residency programs and fellowships that reinforce clinical pharmacologic concepts with practical and real life clinical experiences.[3] With extensive knowledge of pharmacotherapy and the many facets of health care, clinical pharmacists are equipped with the skills necessary to improve outcomes for medical institutions and the patients they serve.

Drug-related morbidity is a significant health care problem. More than 59% of drug-related emergency room visits are preventable,[1] with the most common reasons including adverse drug reactions (39.3%), nonadherence (27.9%), and use of the wrong or suboptimal drug (11.5%).[2] The skills and training that a pharmacist acquired during his or her 4-year didactic training, in addition to another year of clerkship in residency, prepares a pharmacist to serve an essential and complementary role in a health care team.

THE IMPACT OF CLINICAL PHARMACISTS
Improved Clinical Outcomes

Regardless of the health care setting, pharmacists play an active part in improving clinical outcomes and promoting patient safety and cost efficiency. A retrospective study performed in the medical home setting evaluated the impact of clinical pharmacy services (CPS) on diabetes-related clinical outcomes. Results showed that patients receiving care from the pharmacist compared with patients receiving usual care had about a threefold increased likelihood of achieving an A1c less than 7%.[4] Pharmacists evaluated medications, made drug therapy and dose adjustments, monitored adherence, and provided education and follow-up.

Another study validated the positive impact of clinical pharmacists on health outcomes in patients with heart failure. Gattis and colleagues[5] examined the effects of medication evaluations and therapeutic recommendations made by pharmacists on mortality for patients with heart failure and left ventricular dysfunction. Patients who received pharmacist intervention had significantly lower all-cause mortality and heart failure events when compared with the control group. Several other studies have shown similar trends of positive impact on patient care and clinical outcomes with pharmacist interventions.[6–8]

Clinical pharmacist intervention can positively affect adverse drug event rates and prevent medication-related harm. One study examined the effect of pharmacist participation on medical rounds in the intensive care unit. Results showed the rate of preventable adverse drug events was decreased by 66% in the unit with pharmacist participation.[9] A 2-year cross-sectional epidemiologic study assessed the impact of clinical pharmacist oversight of a 180-inpatient bed maternity and children's hospital. The study reported nearly 1500 pharmacist interventions, including correction of over 800 medication-dosing errors of which over 200 cases were clinically serious or potentially fatal.[10] Another prospective, nonrandomized trial of over 500 patients assessed the capacity of a pharmacist-led inpatient anticoagulation service to reduce the incidence of supratherapeutic international normalized ratios (INRs) in patients receiving oral anticoagulation with warfarin. Compared with the control group, which received no pharmacist surveillance, the intervention group had a 77% reduction in rate of over-anticoagulation. Moreover, the intervention group also experienced an overall increase in rates of medication adherence and maintenance of therapeutic INRs.[11] What is evident from such studies is that clinical pharmacist services help decrease the number of adverse drug events and, consequently, health care cost associated with resolving the sequelae of those events.

Economic Impact

Many studies have demonstrated the fiscal benefits of clinical pharmacists for patients as well as patient care facilities. Pharmacist interventions made during patient encounters in hospital emergency rooms can reduce emergency room hospital admissions and improve patient medication adherence with no loss of patients' health-related quality of life and a reduction in health care costs for patients and hospitals.[12]

PHARMACY PRACTICE IN UNITED STATES HEALTH CARE

In many, if not all, states in the United States, clinical pharmacists have established themselves as health care providers in the primary care setting. These pharmacists, also referred to as ambulatory care pharmacists, supplement the efforts of clinicians, such as physicians, nurse practitioners, and physicians' assistants, by providing comprehensive pharmacotherapy management and disease education to patients with diabetes, dyslipidemia, hypertension, and other chronic health issues, including patients with multiple comorbidities. Responsibilities include offering medication reconciliation and medication therapy management services, troubleshooting medication access issues, ordering and reviewing laboratory tests to monitor disease progression, and counseling patients on their medications and disease state goals. These pharmacists may also serve as consultants to other clinicians in the medical office when it comes to drug treatment recommendations. Just how much authority a pharmacist has to work independently should be qualified by clinic policy, as should the referral of patients to pharmacy services (eg, via direct clinician order or prospective chart review and active recruitment).

Even in the community pharmacy retail setting there is a gradual movement toward incorporating similar ambulatory care services in everyday practice. Community pharmacies are collaborating with insurance companies, city and state organizations, physician groups, and other sponsors to provide patients with health care services in the retail setting. These services include health screenings, chronic disease state coaching and management programs, and medication therapy management services. Similar to ambulatory care pharmacists, the prescriptive authority of a pharmacist working in the community retail setting is based on collaborative agreements with physicians.

Programs such as the Health Resources and Services Administration's Patient Safety and Clinical Pharmacy Services Collaborative (PSPC) are helping to advocate for the integration of CPS into a variety of clinic and health care settings nationwide. This organization has recently partnered with the Center for Medicare and Medicaid Services and other quality improvement organizations to assist its PSPC team members in providing safe, evidence-based care and medication management of high-risk, high-cost, complex patients. The organization also works to raise the profile of ambulatory care pharmacists' capabilities and credentials. PSPC teams' activities involve pharmacist efforts at rural health centers, community clinics, schools of pharmacy, and public health departments.[13]

State and Federal Level Involvement

Pharmacists also collaborate with state Boards of Pharmacy and other regulatory agencies to work on changes needed in education and state practice acts to implement patient-focused pharmacy services while maintaining public safety. Examples of these changes include expanding the role of technicians and greater use of health information technology (HIT).

Pharmacists in California spent two decades convincing that state's Board of Pharmacy to allow pharmacy technicians to complete medication cassette fills by other technicians to free time for pharmacists to provide direct patient care.[14] This allowed pharmacists to spend more time on the floor, working with other physicians to reduce medication errors.

Another example of pharmacists currently making state and federal progress is in the area of HIT, which is a technology that has shown to improve patient safety and reduce subsequent harm and injury to patients. The enactment of the Health Information Technology for Economic and Clinical Health (HITECH) Act in 2009 provides financial incentives to physicians and hospitals for the adoption and meaningful use of electronic health records (EHRs).[15] However, pharmacists do not qualify as eligible providers for these incentives, even though many of the current electronic quality measures to verify incentive payments require interoperability with pharmacists as providers.

In spite of this obstacle, pharmacists in the Pharmacy e-Health Information Technology Collaborative have developed a strategic plan to ensure that the use of EHRs supports safe and effective medication use, continuity of care, and access to the patient care services of pharmacists in conjunction with other members of the patient care team.[16] The Collaborative was involved in the development of the Pharmacist/Pharmacy Provider Electronic Health Record (PP-EHR) to support the incentive requirements related to pharmacy services. Pharmacists are engaging in discussions with the Center for Medicare and Medicaid Services, the Office of the National Coordinator, and federal advisory committees as part of a national effort to recommend that pharmacists are recognized as eligible providers of medication-related patient care services and meaningful users of and contributors to EHRs. Clinical pharmacists are developing funding opportunities at the state level for pharmacist-related programs and health information exchanges.

In California, a pharmacy grant program has been developed to support the adoption of electronic prescribing among independent pharmacies.[17] The California Department of Health and Human Services will establish a train-the-trainer program to provide technical support in electronic prescribing for community pharmacies in California.[18] The program will be administered through a HIT curriculum that can be taught in a standardized and consistent format across schools of pharmacy in California. To broaden the reach of the HIT program, curriculum reform will expand beyond schools of pharmacy to facilitate interdisciplinary HIT education with other health professional schools (ie, schools of medicine and nursing). This program is developed to be sustainable with the training programs continuing well beyond the duration of funding under HITECH.

PATIENT-CENTERED MEDICAL HOME

The patient-centered medical home (PCMH) model aims to "deliver structured and coordinated care that meets the specific needs of each patient."[19] Care is provided through a multidisciplinary approach: the collaboration of the patient, the physician, and other health care providers practicing at the top of their license and integrated into the PCMH team. In anticipation of the positive outcomes of this model, the Institute of Medicine (IOM) has incorporated the PCMH model into the education of future physicians to prepare for an easy transition into this new primary care model.[20,21] This redefined role can potentially maximize the quality and coordination of care, as well as achieve cost reduction.[22]

Inclusion of a clinical pharmacist into the PCMH model can serve many benefits as health care costs continue to escalate and medication management in patients with chronic diseases becomes increasingly complex. First, pharmacists are equipped with the expertise to address appropriate and cost-effective medication use and prevent medication-related problems. A study by Ernst and Grizzle[23] found that the mean cost of medical problems from drug therapy (eg, adverse side effects, hospitalizations, over-prescribing, nonadherence) is $1105 per incident. Using a clinical pharmacist as part of the PCMH can reduce the financial burden by detecting and resolving medication-related issues through the delivery of services such as Medication Therapy Management (MTM). Many other health care systems, such as Kaiser and Veterans Affairs, have already realized the value of a clinical pharmacist in this capacity and have included them as part of the health care team.

Clinical pharmacists possess expertise on optimization, safety, and effectiveness of medication use and can assist in modifying drug therapy regimens. Primary care providers will often refer patients to specialists for medication adjustments (eg, worsening diabetes to an endocrinologist). However, having a clinical pharmacist as part of the team is a cost-effective choice for medication changes. In safety net clinics in the greater Los Angeles area, CPS provided to a diabetic, underserved population with A1cs greater than 9%, showed a clinically and statistically significant decrease in A1c of 1.48%.[4] Additionally, pharmacists are increasingly accessible and can spend time with patients that the physician cannot commit to because of scheduling constraints.

As part of a larger University of California, Los Angeles (UCLA) Health System practice redesign initiative, a clinical pharmacist has been incorporated into the health care team at UCLA Department of Family Medicine's UCLA Family Health Center (UFHC) and is working with physicians and a family nurse practitioner to help high-risk patients with uncontrolled diabetes meet their clinical outcome goals. According to NCQA,[22] one of the key elements of the PCMH is the enhanced access to health care providers to ensure continuity of care. A patient's appointment with the pharmacist is usually scheduled in between physician follow-up visits to address any medication-related problems. For the initial visit, patients are instructed to bring in all their medications including over-the-counter medications as well as herbal supplements. The clinical pharmacist then performs a comprehensive assessment of proper medication use and identifies medication-related problems that may interfere with patients' meeting their individualized treatment goals. Many issues are identified, including nonadherence due to insurance constraints, refill issues, accessibility to the prescribing physician, and/or unclear directions for use. During the initial assessment, the clinical pharmacist may also uncover the patient's current and historical experience with medications. These experiences reflect the patient's beliefs and reveal concerns and expectations about his or her medications, which may affect medication adherence. After the reasons for nonadherence are identified, the clinical pharmacist will use motivational interviewing techniques to engage patients to positively move toward their intended outcomes. Many of these techniques are used to involve patients in developing an individualized action plan at each visit, which is then relayed to all other health care professionals on the PCMH team through an MTM consultation note via encrypted email. Communication of these clinical pharmacy interventions is delivered to all team members involved in the patient's care, including the primary care physician, the family nurse practitioner, dietician, clinical psychologist, and subspecialty consultants. The MTM clinic note records all interventions made by the clinical pharmacist, including drug initiations, therapeutic substitutions, medication discontinuations, and patient education efforts, as well as referrals made, laboratory results, and vaccinations ordered.

Although a reimbursement model does not currently exist, clinical pharmacist services at UFHC are billed using E&M code 99211, in which a physician reviews and signs off on all interventions documented and made by the pharmacist. Additionally, the time spent with patients during each visit is tracked using CPT Codes 99607, 99606, 99605.

In a short 2 months, the impact of CPS at UFHC has already been realized. Improvements in blood pressure, increased medication adherence, reduction in out-of-pocket costs for medications, and increased patient and provider satisfaction have only been a few of the outcomes achieved.

BARRIERS TO SUCCESSFUL IMPLEMENTATION OF CPS

Implementation of CPS, whether in the community, ambulatory, or inpatient setting, can be difficult for a variety of reasons. The value of CPS has been clearly demonstrated in numerous publications in the literature, but each patient-care setting seeking to establish CPS may present a unique set of challenges to achieve this goal.

Financial Constraints

One of the most significant barriers to establishing CPS is the challenge of securing funding to support the service. Pharmacists' salaries may start upwards of $90,000 annually and these wages (benefits and other overhead notwithstanding) add to the already high cost of labor within health care delivery systems. Owing to current medical billing standards, it may be difficult to recuperate these expenditures in revenue generated from patient encounters, medication therapy management, or other nondispensing services. Under current Medicare legislation (Medicare Prescription Drug, Improvement and Modernization Act of 2003), pharmacists are not designated as health care providers and, consequently, are not eligible to receive compensation for their clinical and pharmaceutical care services under Medicare Part B. Insurance plans nationwide (both private and public) have simulated this billing model and have disallowed reimbursement for pharmacists acting in this role. Also, unlike other health care professionals, pharmacists typically do not collect professional fees for their services. There are some states in the United States that have passed laws allowing pharmacists to charge for services rendered (as opposed to simply billing for products; ie, dispensed medications) but these states are in the minority and pharmacists must negotiate reimbursement rates on a per-payer, per-employer, or per-benefits manager basis.[24] Some CPS programs support themselves with fees resulting from associated medication dispensing services,[24,25] but not all pharmacy departments are set up to support this business model. Moreover, as prescription reimbursement rates decline, it becomes more difficult for this dwindling revenue source to cover all the expenses related to CPS activities and personnel.[26]

Given these lack of opportunities for revenue generation, it can be challenging for pharmacy services to promote themselves as cost-neutral.[26] Establishment of pharmacy services, therefore, typically necessitates a plan for sustainability via cost avoidance or cost-efficiency measures.[26] Financial analyses of existing clinical pharmacy programs have shown the benefit of a pharmacist in lowering drug costs, reducing medication errors, preventing adverse drug reactions and their subsequent medical management, and/or shortening lengths of hospital stays.[27–29] Administrators may remain skeptical, however, of whether that evidence would justify establishment of CPS at their particular institution.[27] Review studies or other literature demonstrating evidence of benefit-to-cost ratios of CPS may not be applicable at the local level where decisions are made.[29,30] Other issues, including an inflexible budget, political objectives, and lack of time or resources to do an institution-specific prospective economic or feasibility evaluation, may also preclude validation of implementation of CPS.[30]

Demonstrating Need

Apart from the financial concerns listed above, CPS must also be able to prove its value to its stakeholders. Such proof includes demonstrating an ability to improve clinical outcomes, patient satisfaction, and quality of life indicators. Relying on these measures alone as justification for CPS can be thorny, however, because a health care entity typically is already striving to promote patient advocacy and meet these objectives.[26]

To determine how CPS will make the largest impact within a particular patient care environment, it is imperative that a needs assessment be done. The pharmacist may review medical charts to see what types of patients are seen (eg, number of medications they take, comorbidities), the types of medication errors committed, and how successful the practice is at reaching treatment goals. The needs may be specific to each practice site, or even specific to different departments within one site (eg, family medicine department vs emergency department vs intensive care unit).

Health care providers and administrators may not know what CPS is or what a clinic pharmacist does, or they may think that other health professionals at lower cost could perform these pharmacy services. Although Medicare Part D will pay its plans for medication therapy management services, the plans are not specifically required to use pharmacists in this role.[24] A needs assessment would hopefully reveal which drug-related services may already be performed by other departments and health team members. Regrettably, if a service offered by CPS is viewed as duplicative, it may fail because of existing allegiance to the established service.[25]

Organizational Issues

Each practice setting may present unique challenges for implementation of CPS. In the community or retail pharmacy, for example, patients may not recognize their pharmacist as a service provider. They may not even feel compelled to interact with the pharmacist at each visit to the pharmacy. Community pharmacists also lack access to their patients' complete medical records; therefore, providing comprehensive medication therapy management or other forms of CPS may be problematic or potentially viewed as unsafe.

In the hospital setting, the pharmacy department will need administrators' buy-in before taking steps to establish CPS. As these senior leaders measure up the financial standing of their organization against other organizations, the department's budget (consisting of labor and drug costs) may be tightly controlled and relatively inflexible in accommodating the expense of CPS.[31] Literature detailing CPS achievements at other sites might not convince executive leadership that the success is reproducible at their own institution. Often, hospitals are built to house centralized pharmacy infrastructure only (eg, a basement-level dispensary) and may not be able to accommodate satellite offices for CPS personnel. Also, discontinuous and rotating physician services may make it difficult for pharmacists to build rapport with their colleagues.[27]

Cultural Acceptance

The profession of pharmacy has evolved through the years. The traditional tasks of manufacturing, compounding, order entry, and drug distribution are gradually being supplanted by responsibilities of patient consultation, clinical services, and pharmaceutical care.[32,33] Certain health care providers may not yet recognize the expanded role pharmacists can play in patient care and, lamentably, may show a lack of enthusiasm for pharmacist's participation in collaborative, interdisciplinary care efforts.[27] Usually a physician champion or support from an administrator is needed from the outset to advocate for CPS as a valuable and necessary service.

The integration of CPS within the UFHC has been widely accepted and welcomed by the practice and the clinical pharmacist is viewed as a valuable member of the PCMH team.

SOLUTIONS

The role of pharmacists as members of the health care team continues to expand beyond conventional medication dispensing in the United States. As mentioned, there is substantial evidence that CPS is directly associated with decreased mortality, fewer complications, lower hospital charges, and a significant reduction in preventable adverse drug events among hospitalized patients.[9,34,35] This is consistent with the American College of Clinical Pharmacists vision for which "pharmacists will be recognized and valued as the preeminent health care professionals responsible for the use of medicines in the prevention and treatment of disease" and function at the top of their level of training and skill.[36]

With a projected shortage of primary care providers, there is an unprecedented opportunity for well-trained, underutilized clinical pharmacists to expand access to care in the areas of chronic disease management and preventative medicine. State and/or federal regulations that require integration of pharmacists into the health care team, access to medical records, and changes to the reimbursement model to support CPS will lead to pharmacists practicing at the top of their training and improving patient care.

Reimbursement Models for Clinical Pharmacy Services

Despite evidence that CPS improves patient outcomes and provides a positive return-on-investment, reimbursement models have progressed slowly.[37–39] There is currently no single model; therefore, pharmacists should be acquainted with all the various models of payment. These include direct payment (fee-for-service), indirect payment (eg, payment to the physician, who in turn pays the pharmacist), cost reduction (CPS are justified based on the amount of money saved), payment (ie, salary) by a health care system for value added and improvement in patient care outcomes, capitation (payment per person per month), and performance-based payment (payment bonus based on achieving a target).[40] In general, securing payment for CPS has been difficult partly because pharmacists are not designated as providers under Medicare Part B. Therefore, obtaining Part B provider status should remain a primary goal to ensure payment for services and to gain necessary recognition of pharmacists as medication therapy managers.

The inclusion of pharmacist-delivered services and the shift to team-based care in the Affordable Care Act is promising.[41] Under this regulation, there is an opportunity to establish a standard for widespread payment for clinical services. Pharmacists should also stay actively engaged in the discussions regarding the provisions under the Affordable Care Act to ensure appropriate reimbursements are applied to valued services. It is a critical time to do so because the reimbursement structures by most major payers are changing.[42] The margins gained from prescription dispensing are declining and will not be sufficient for clinical services rendered by pharmacists.

There is also an opportunity for pharmacists and their associations to make incremental progress by negotiating with payers on reimbursement for specific sets of services. Currently, health insurance companies, pharmacy benefit management companies, medical groups, employers, city or county governments, and state Medicaid agencies pay for clinical services by pharmacists, such as MTM, smoking cessation, asthma management, lipid control, and diabetes management. Studies, such as the one conducted in Minnesota, demonstrate that pharmacists working in collaboration with primary care providers identified and resolved drug therapy problems, which lead to improved clinical outcomes and reduced overall health expenditures.[43] Although implementation of pay-for-performance and pay-for-quality systems remains a challenge, the value-based purchasing of MTM services appeals to employers and payers. The appeal relates to competing on results and improving quality in health care by achieving goals of therapy.

Documentation for CPS

Documentation is an essential component of providing CPS. It is necessary to record the nature of the encounter, the patient problems identified, and the follow-up plans. The format of the document varies between institutions, although national organizations have offered standards for community practice.[44] The documentation serves as evidence of continuity of care between the patient, the pharmacist, and the primary care provider. Appropriate documentation is critically important for accurate reimbursement for services rendered by the pharmacist. To successfully initiate claims, pharmacists must assure that documented is presented concisely, legibly, and accurately. The documentation also must correspond to the level of services rendered.[45]

Recommendations for Immediate Call to Action

Many studies have demonstrated the beneficial impact of pharmacist-provided care in the areas of therapeutic, safety, and humanistic outcomes.[46] Yet, the vision of the pharmacist role within a PCMH-centered medical home practice has not been fully realized. Pharmacists and organizations should continue to use the substantial evidence to promote stakeholders' understanding, recognition, and use of CPS to increase use of pharmacists as members of the health care team and as direct patient-care providers. Achieving this vision will require well-coordinated efforts that include gaining support of health care administrations and members of the various professional associations by demonstrating the impact of CPS on improving quality and safety of patient care, improving patient satisfaction, and achieving cost savings.

To achieve recognition among other members of the health care team, the health system requires the director of pharmacy to perform at a proactive executive level using a systems-based approach to assist the health system in meeting its strategic goals and objectives. The director or pharmacy manager can justify CPS by providing the substantial evidence that has been published in past and current literature. Although a local evaluation will require resources and may delay the implementation of CPS, it might be an important and necessary step to improve the understanding of the value-added competent that well-trained clinical pharmacists can provide to patients and the organization. Pharmacy executives will need to understand and use the basic model of evaluation, which includes consideration of both costs and outcomes, and inclusion of a comparator group.[29]

Health care settings should increase availability of and access to medication management services provided by pharmacists in a team-based approach. The specific roles should be clearly defined and transparent to all members of the health care team. A stepwise approach to the development and implementation of CPS can facilitate the expansion of these services across an integrated health system. The favorable impact of CPS in ambulatory clinic systems has been demonstrated and was based on establishing the following key components:

- A successful model of care in a university hospital setting and subsequent adaptation to the model to meet the needs of a community hospital
- A standardized billing process that facilitates appropriate distribution of revenue to pharmacy cost centers across the health system
- Collaborative agreements with clinical pharmacists to improve medication therapy outcomes
- Improved continuity of care and patient outcomes.[47]

Improving patient care outcomes is achieved through communication, collaboration, and coordination of care between various health care professionals in all health care practice settings. The foundation of this patient-centered model approach includes the recognition of pharmacists as drug therapy experts and, therefore, as members of the health care team who provide a unique set of knowledge and skills. The clinical pharmacist has been trained as an objective, evidence-based source of therapeutic information to proactively ensure safe and effective use of medications. Routine clinical interventions and recommendations involve interaction with patients and health professionals on a regular basis.

SUMMARY

Pharmacists in all sectors (eg, outpatient primary care, community health centers hospitals, skilled nursing facilities) have been highly underutilized and only recently has the profession been encouraged and commended to practice at the top of their license. As these opportunities to advance the profession evolve, pharmacists must collectively rise to the occasion and work collaboratively to help patients and physicians positively and more efficiently move toward better health outcomes through comprehensive medication therapy management.

REFERENCES

1. Winterstein AG, et al. Preventable drug-related hospital admissions. Ann Pharmacother 2002;36(7–8):1238–48.
2. Zed PJ, et al. Incidence, severity and preventability of medication-related visits to the emergency department: a prospective study. CMAJ 2008;178(12): 1563–9.
3. Burke JM, et al. Clinical pharmacist competencies. Pharmacotherapy 2008;28(6): 806–15.
4. Johnson KA, et al. The impact of clinical pharmacy services integrated into medical homes on diabetes-related clinical outcomes. Ann Pharmacother 2010; 44(12):1877–86.
5. Gattis WA, et al. Reduction in heart failure events by the addition of a clinical pharmacist to the heart failure management team: results of the Pharmacist in Heart Failure Assessment Recommendation and Monitoring (PHARM) Study. Arch Intern Med 1999;159(16):1939–45.

6. Chisholm-Burns MA, et al. Impact of clinical pharmacy services on renal transplant recipients' adherence and outcomes. Patient Prefer Adherence 2008;2:287–92.

7. Cording MA, et al. Development of a pharmacist-managed lipid clinic. Ann Pharmacother 2002;36(5):892–904.

8. Kiel PJ, McCord AD. Pharmacist impact on clinical outcomes in a diabetes disease management program via collaborative practice. Ann Pharmacother 2005;39(11):1828–32.

9. Leape LL, et al. Pharmacist participation on physician rounds and adverse drug events in the intensive care unit. JAMA 1999;282(3):267–70.

10. Fernandez-Llamazares CM, et al. Impact of clinical pharmacist interventions in reducing paediatric prescribing errors. Arch Dis Child 2012;97(6):564–8.

11. Dawson NL, et al. Inpatient warfarin management: pharmacist management using a detailed dosing protocol. J Thromb Thrombolysis 2012;33(2):178–84.

12. Desborough JA, et al. A cost-consequences analysis of an adherence focused pharmacist-led medication review service. Int J Pharm Pract 2012;20(1):41–9.

13. HRSA.gov. [cited 2012 April 4]. Available at: http://www.hrsa.gov/publichealth/clinical/patientsafety/pspc4_overview.pdf.

14. Topics D. California accepts 'Tech-Check-Tech' in hospitals. 2006 [cited 2012].

15. Register F. Rules and regulations. October 30, 2009.

16. Collaborative P.e.-H.I.T. Roadmap for Pharmacy Health Information Technology Integration in U.S. Health Care.

17. eConnect C. ePrescribing Advisory Group Meeting. 2012.

18. Services. D.o.H.C. California State Medi-Cal Health Information Technology Plan.

19. Crosby J, GP, Rogers E. The Patient-Centered Medical Home: Integrating Comprehensive Medication Management to Optimize Patient Outcomes (A Resource Guide) P.C.P.C.C. (PCPCC), Editor 2005.

20. Erickson S, Hambleton J. A pharmacy's journey toward the patient-centered medical home. J Am Pharm Assoc (2003) 2011;51(2):156–60.

21. Peterson C. Health professions education: a bridge to quality. Tar Heel Nurse 2003;65(4):12.

22. Abrons JP, Smith M. Patient-centered medical homes: primer for pharmacists. J Am Pharm Assoc (2003) 2011;51(3):e38–48 [quiz: e49–50].

23. Ernst FR, Grizzle AJ. Drug-related morbidity and mortality: updating the cost-of-illness model. J Am Pharm Assoc (Wash) 2001;41(2):192–9.

24. Stubbings J, et al. Payment for clinical pharmacy services revisited. Pharmacotherapy 2011;31(1):1–8.

25. Harris IM, et al. Developing a business-practice model for pharmacy services in ambulatory settings. Pharmacotherapy 2008;28(2):285.

26. Dole EJ, Murawski MM. Reimbursement for clinical services provided by pharmacists: what are we doing wrong? Am J Health Syst Pharm 2007;64(1):104–6.

27. Curtiss FR, Wertheimer AI. A project to implement clinical pharmacy practice in rural environments. Public Health Rep 1978;93(1):41–5.

28. Hughes DW, Roth JM, Laurel Y. Establishing emergency department clinical pharmacy services. Am J Health Syst Pharm 2010;67(13):1053–7.

29. Anderson SV, Schumock GT. Evaluation and justification of clinical pharmacy services. Expert Rev Pharmacoecon Outcomes Res 2009;9(6):539–45.

30. De Rijdt T, Willems L, Simoens S. Hospital pharmacists versus hospital administrators: a struggle for clinical pharmacy services. Expert Rev Pharmacoecon Outcomes Res 2009;9(6):497–8.

31. Knoer S. Surviving and thriving in tough economic times. Am J Health Syst Pharm 2010;67(23):2000, 2002, 2004.

32. Holland RW, Nimmo CM. Transitions, part 1: beyond pharmaceutical care. Am J Health Syst Pharm 1999;56(17):1758–64.
33. Pickette SG, Muncey L, Wham D. Implementation of a standard pharmacy clinical practice model in a multihospital system. Am J Health Syst Pharm 2010;67(9): 751–6.
34. Bond CA, Raehl CL, Franke T. Interrelationships among mortality rates, drug costs, total cost of care, and length of stay in United States hospitals: summary and recommendations for clinical pharmacy services and staffing. Pharmacotherapy 2001;21(2):129–41.
35. Bond CA, Raehl CL. Clinical pharmacy services, pharmacy staffing, and hospital mortality rates. Pharmacotherapy 2007;27(4):481–93.
36. Guglielmo BJ. A prescription for improved chronic disease management: have community pharmacists function at the top of their training: comment on "Engaging physicians and pharmacists in providing smoking cessation counseling." Arch Intern Med 2010;170(18):1646–7.
37. Perez A, et al. ACCP: economic evaluations of clinical pharmacy services: 2001-2005. Pharmacotherapy 2009;29(1):128.
38. Schumock GT, et al. Evidence of the economic benefit of clinical pharmacy services: 1996-2000. Pharmacotherapy 2003;23(1):113–32.
39. Elenbaas RM, Worthen DB. Transformation of a profession: an overview of the 20th century. Pharm Hist 2009;51(4):151–82.
40. Nutescu EA, Klotz RS. Basic terminology in obtaining reimbursement for pharmacists' cognitive services. Am J Health Syst Pharm 2007;64(2):186–92.
41. Lipton HL. Pharmacists and health reform: go for it! Pharmacotherapy 2010; 30(10):967–72.
42. Patient Protection and Affordable Care Act, HR 3590, 111. [cited 2010 September 24]. Available at: http://democrats.senate.gov/reform/patient-protection-affordable-care-act-as-passed.pdf.
43. Isetts BJ, et al. Clinical and economic outcomes of medication therapy management services: the Minnesota experience. J Am Pharm Assoc (2003) 2008;48(2): 203–11, 3 p following 211.
44. Stores A.P.A.a.t.N.A.o.C.D. Medication therapy management in community pharmacy practiced: core elements of an MTM service. [cited 2007 July 27]. Available at: http://www.aphanet.org/.
45. American Pharmacists Association, National Association of Chain Drug Stores Foundation. Medication Therapy Management in community pharmacy practice: core elements of an MTM service (version 1.0). J Am Pharm Assoc (2003) 2005; 45(5):573–9.
46. Chisholm-Burns MA, et al. US pharmacists' effect as team members on patient care: systematic review and meta-analyses. Med Care 2010;48(10):923–33.
47. Epplen K, et al. Stepwise approach to implementing ambulatory clinical pharmacy services. Am J Health Syst Pharm 2007;64(9):945–51.

Palliative Care in the Patient-Centered Medical Home

David J. Wallenstein, MD

KEYWORDS

- Hierarchical condition categories • Palliative care • Patient-centered medical home
- Population management • Physician orders for life-sustaining treatment
- Risk factor value

KEY POINTS

- There are presently few published data on the delivery of palliative care services in the outpatient setting and virtually no published data on either the integration of palliative care into primary care practice or its applicability to innovative models of health care delivery, such as the patient-centered medical home and accountable care organizations.
- New topics for health services delivery research are suggested. Because of the lack of data, this article draws on information collected from inpatient palliative care delivery and includes anecdotal experiences from the outpatient pain medicine and palliative care clinic of an academic department of family medicine.

PALLIATIVE CARE: WHAT IT IS AND WHAT IT IS NOT

A useful working definition of palliative care as a medical discipline is that put forth by Diane Meier, MD, at Mount Sinai Medical Center in Manhattan:

Palliative care is specialized medical care for people with serious illnesses. This type of care is focused on providing patients with the symptoms, pain and stress of a serious illness – whatever the diagnosis. The goal is to improve the quality of life for both the patient and the family. Palliative care is provided by a team of doctors, nurses and other specialists who work with a patient's other doctors to provide an extra layer of support. Palliative care is appropriate at any age and at any stage in a serious illness, and can be provided together with curative treatment.[1]

There are 3 salient points to be gleaned from Meier's definition: (1) palliative care and hospice care, which is specialized care for people at the end of life, are not synonymous, and admission to a hospice program is not necessarily a goal of palliative care; (2) palliative care can be provided at the same time as disease-modifying and curative treatments, as well as to patients after curative treatment who have no evidence of disease but have residual pain and symptom issues; and (3) palliative care provides an extra layer of support to patients with serious and life-limiting illnesses, their

Department of Family Medicine, UCLA, CA, USA
E-mail address: dwallenstein@mednet.ucla.edu

Prim Care Clin Office Pract 39 (2012) 627–631
http://dx.doi.org/10.1016/j.pop.2012.08.009   **primarycare.theclinics.com**

families, and also their health care providers, but it is not intended to take the place of primary care. The importance of palliative medicine within the context of primary care has been recognized. The American Board of Family Medicine has provided 2 pathways toward a Certificate of Added Qualifications (CAQ). One pathway, which has been available to board-certified physicians from 2008 to 2012, is a board examination, after which further training requirements are necessary. According to the American Board of Family Medicine, this board, in a joint venture with the American Board of Internal Medicine and 8 other American Board of Medical Specialty boards, offers a CAQ in hospice and palliative medicine. This CAQ is designated to recognize excellence among certified family physicians who emphasize the care of seriously ill and dying patients with life-limiting illnesses in their practice.[1]

In clinical practice, palliative care consists of 2 general areas of focus: (1) providing the patient with meticulous pain and symptom management, including attention to mental health issues, and (2) supporting and facilitating the patient and the patient's family in identifying and implementing realistic goals of care. To provide optimal benefit to patients and their families, palliative care properly involves itself at an earlier point in the disease trajectory than does hospice care.

In the inpatient, acute care setting, multiple studies have shown that palliative care improves the quality of life for patients with serious, complex illnesses and their family members, often saving millions of dollars annually in downstream costs, and frequently increasing the efficiency of the primary care physicians and other specialists managing these extremely ill patients. Taking this concept a step further, embedding palliative care within a primary care patient-centered medical home (PCMH) with innovative strategies in health care delivery systems has been under way for several years at University of California, Los Angeles, and research to tease out the impact is forthcoming.

ADVANCING AGE, CHRONIC DISEASE, AND SOARING COSTS

By 2050, the proportion of the population older than 65 years is projected to more than double. As people age, they develop a multiplicity of chronic illnesses, which not only results in increased health care services and cost but increases the complexity of the decisions that they, and their decision makers, confront regarding treatment options, comfort, life-sustaining interventions, and end-of-life decisions. According to Willard and Bodenheimer,[2] patients with 5 or more chronic conditions accounted for 76% of Medicare spending in 2002, and average spending for these patients is 17 times higher than for patients without chronic conditions.

Outpatient physicians with additional qualifications in palliative care training may be ideally suited to facilitate the health care team in addressing patients' preferences for end-of-life treatment, but data are limited. Lee and colleagues found that for 58 advanced directives that used the Physician Orders for Life-Sustaining Treatment document, do not resuscitate (DNR) or other levels of care such as comfort care and limited, advanced, or full intervention were performed for those with DNR orders for 91% of the patients but only at the level specified in only 25 cases or 46% for other levels of care.[3] Seriously ill patients are often subjected to burdensome, medically inappropriate, futile treatments earlier in the trajectory of disease, not just at the end of life, the default choice when patients' preferences for care are unknown.

Pending further research and evaluation, our patients and their families who have been referred to and treated within our outpatient academic family medicine PCMH have indicated a high level of satisfaction. From preliminary data, access to a physician specialist with expertise in pain and symptom management likely shows increases in both patient comfort and quality of life and a decrease in acute care hospital admissions and emergency room use for this at-risk population.

Implementation of models of health care delivery such as the PCMH, particularly with the phasing in of provisions of the Affordable Healthcare Act, brings more patients who can benefit from palliative care services into the ambulatory medicine setting. Inpatient palliative care consultation has tended to occur in the setting of acute clinical deterioration, catastrophic events or injury, and at the end of life. Including palliative care consultation in high-volume PCMH increases access to these services to patients in less acute and emergent circumstances. Furthermore, many of those who benefit from the integration of palliative care services into the ambulatory clinic are patients with evolving multisystem dysfunction and debility, a large demographic who surely benefit from ongoing goals of care discussion, advanced directive review and revision, and appropriate pain and symptom management.

Increasingly, health care delivery occurs with emphasis on cost-effectiveness, outcome measures supporting provision of high-quality, evidence-based, medically appropriate treatment, and provider accountability, by both private payers and by entitlements. Palliative care, with its dual focus on pain and symptom management and goals of care discussion and planning, is well positioned to facilitate the inclusion of these mandates into outpatient primary care. Furthermore, there is some evidence to suggest that including palliative care specialists in a medical practice setting increases the productivity of the providers and positively affects practice revenue.

In our academic PCMH family medicine practice, we have treated patients with complex, life-limiting illnesses complicated by psychiatric and chemical dependency comorbidities. Input and access to other specialists in addiction and behavior medicine, psychiatry, and social work (all in a single location) have facilitated an organized and structured approach to the management of these challenging, often chaotic clinical scenarios.

CASE EXAMPLE: PRINCIPLES OF THE PCMH WITHIN AN ACADEMIC FAMILY MEDICINE OUTPATIENT CENTER WITH AN EMBEDDED PAIN MEDICINE AND PALLIATIVE CARE CLINIC

Mr X was a 70-year-old married man, father of 2 and an immigrant from southeast Asia. His history was significant for a history of prostate cancer, long-standing, poorly controlled diabetes and hypertension, worsening chronic kidney disease, cognitive impairment, and intermittent paranoid ideation. Realizing that Mr X's cognitive impairment was worsening, the primary care physician and the patient's family had attempted to discuss advanced directives and preferences for treatment, but this resulted in a rift between Mr X and his primary care physician as well as family discord at the patient's home that required the local police to be summoned. Based on multiple factors, a referral from the family physician to the pain medicine and palliative care working with the family medicine PCMH to provide complex care was requested to address the patient's upper body pain and paresthesia, which were difficult to control, and his complicated home situation.

In the months before his referral, Mr X had been hospitalized multiple times for severe constipation with a small bowel obstruction, altered mental status, and acute or chronic renal failure: all conditions secondary to medication nonadherence. With permission from the patient, a discussion with family members revealed that Mr X believed that his pain was untreatable and refused to take prescribed pain medications because he found the side effects (somnolence and constipation) untenable. Although the referring physician considered the patient's pain might be a result of a metastatic prostate cancer, the patient declined any workup to address the possibility of this condition.

During follow-up visits with the palliative care physician, care was coordinated with the primary care physician and other health care team members, including home health nursing, to evaluate barriers to care. A pain management regime that relieved pain without causing somnolence and worsening confusion along with a bowel regime to prevent constipation was instituted. After several months of improved medication adherence for pain and symptom management, Mr X developed a sense of trust with his palliative care physician, agreed to participate in a family discussion on goals of care, and advanced directives were completed.

Mr X continued to be followed in his medical home for the next 3 years, and during that time, was hospitalized only twice: once for altered mental status related to a urinary tract infection (his advanced directive stated that he would agree to a trial of intravenous [IV] antibiotics but would not wish transfer to a critical care setting or to undergo resuscitation) and once for community-acquired pneumonia (again, his advanced directives allowed a trial of IV antibiotic treatment). However, his quality of life was relatively high, per his own reports, as well as the reports of his family and he was able to travel to his native country on several occasions.

Shortly after his final trip to his homeland, Mr X became paranoid, with homicidal ideation, and was hospitalized. The primary health care team (consisting of the palliative care doctor, psychiatrist, primary care physician, and clinical pharmacist) worked together to alter the pain management regime to minimize drug-drug interactions between the pain medications and mood-stabilizing medications, and Mr X was able to return home with in-home services.

Six weeks later, Mr X was taken to the emergency department with acute-onset dyspnea and was noted by laboratory tests and electrocardiography to have suffered an ST segment elevation myocardial infarction, resulting in cardiogenic shock and severe pulmonary edema. His advance directive stated that he would not wish either intensive care or any other life-prolonging treatment, but would want comfort-focused care aimed at making his last hours as peaceful as possible. Plans were made to transfer the patient to home hospice care, but he abruptly entered the actively dying phase and died peacefully in the emergency room with his family at his bedside.

MOVING FORWARD: BUILDING FROM SUCCESSFUL PRACTICE IMPROVEMENT

As our academic primary care PCMH evolves through practice redesign, our ability to more efficiently identify seriously ill patient populations at the health system level as well as the practice level will increase. Data have been provided to the practice that include individual patient demographics linked to the patient's primary care physician. Additional information provides the hierarchical condition categories obtained from billing documents such as the summative risk factor value, admission and discharge data, emergency room use, and the percent arrival at outpatient clinical services. This information can determine which patients would most likely benefit from palliative care interventions, creating a patient panel size so that our palliative care physician can manage patients effectively. In addition to the other members of the health care team mentioned earlier, in-office resources consisting of a care coordinator and family nurse practitioner will be used as well as outside community-based services with expertise to support palliative patients. Further, to improve our performance, data will be collected, aggregated, analyzed, and used to make informed decisions about which value metrics will show the highest return on investment. Access to palliative medicine will be expanded to meet the needs of the anticipated increase in seniors and persons with disabilities. A palliative medicine fellowship was launched in July 2012, with plans to increase the number of fellows in July 2013.

REFERENCES

1. Available at: aging.senate.gov/events/hr247gc.pdf, Statement by Gail Austin Cooney, MD FAAHPM, Associate Medical. Accessed August 2012. United States Senate Committee on Aging.
2. Willard R, Bodenheimer T. Available at: http://www.chcf.org/publications/2012/04/building-blocks-primary-care. The building blocks of high-performing primary care: lessons from the field. Accessed April 2012.
3. Garas N, Pantilat S. Advance planning for end-of-life care. Available at: http://www.ahrq.gov/clinic/ptsafety/chap49.htm. Accessed June 2012.

Health Information Technology
Medical Record Documentation Issues in the Electronic Era

Bill Dacey, MHA, MBA, CPC, CPC-I[a],*, Michelle Anne Bholat, MD, MPH[b,c]

KEYWORDS

- Cloning • Medical necessity • Auditing • Quality

KEY POINTS

- Although there are benefits for implementing EHRs as part of the desire of a practice or institution to build patient-centered medical homes, there are also downside risks.
- The intersection of how a practice or institution collects and reports quality metrics using health information technology and subsequently submits claims for services rendered has created unforeseen challenges for which leadership must be aware and address proactively.

THE REGULATORY PROGRESSION

From the passage of the Health Insurance Portability and Accountability Act (HIPAA) legislation in 1996, to the Affordable Care Act in 2010, and the current rush to create accountable care organizations, the side effects of well-intentioned legislation represent an increasing burden on physicians and practices. For most primary care providers this is largely embodied in various aspects of their electronic health record (EHR), although there is plenty of additional work in the faxes, forms, texts, or Google searches to perform what were once simple functions.

Simple is the key word, because it was Title II of HIPAA, known as the "administrative simplification" provision, that required the establishment of national standards for electronic health care transactions. The intent was to reduce redundancy and make claims processing easier. The administrative simplification provisions also began to address the security and privacy of health data. Those standards were meant to improve the efficiency and effectiveness of the health care system by encouraging the widespread use of electronic data interchange in the health care system.

That was the first big step down the electronic path for providers, and vendors and clearinghouses that filed claims for providers handled much of the work. Claims used

[a] The Dacey Group, Inc., 873 Wisconsin Avenue, Palm Harbor, FL 34683, USA; [b] Department of Family Medicine, UCLA, 10-333 Le Conte Avenue, Los Angeles, CA, USA; [c] Center for Health Sciences, 14-143A, Los Angeles, CA 90095–1683, USA
* Corresponding author.
E-mail address: Bill@Daceygroup.com

Prim Care Clin Office Pract 39 (2012) 633–642
http://dx.doi.org/10.1016/j.pop.2012.08.001
0095-4543/12/$ – see front matter © 2012 Published by Elsevier Inc.

to be mailed from the practice. Simplification in this regard was more about efficiency than simplicity.

Next, Subtitle D of the Health Information Technology for Economic and Clinical Health Act, enacted as part of the American Recovery and Reinvestment Act of 2009 (ARRA), addressed the privacy and security concerns associated with the electronic transmission of health information. This extended the privacy and security provisions of HIPAA to business associates of covered entities, including newly updated civil and criminal penalties to business associates. There are now breach (of privacy or security) notification requirements. This imposes new notification requirements on covered entities, business associates, vendors of personal health records, and related entities if a breach of unsecured protected health information occurs. In 2009, the Department of Health and Human Services issued guidance on how to secure protected health information appropriately.

It is unclear why and how electronic communications and storage became so closely intertwined with enhanced privacy and security. Granted, in the case of another Hurricane Katrina we would not have as many medical records floating in the gulf because they will be on a server in the Nevada desert. However, hacking and e-crime is on an equal pace with legitimate software development. If it is all so secure and private, why now do we have such an emphasis on breaches and penalties?

Now that HIPPA has everyone communicating electronically, ARRA includes provisions to promote the meaningful use of health information technology to improve the quality and value of health care. These provisions are set forth in the Health Information Technology for Economic and Clinical Health Act. The ARRA appropriates a total of $2 billion in discretionary funding, in addition to incentive payments under the Medicare and Medicaid programs for providers' adoption and meaningful use of certified EHR technology.

This leads to the current environment of incentive payments for the use of EHRs. Most practices are in the process of working through the initial stages of obtaining payment for meaningful use. One can also mention e-prescribing, PQRS (Physician Quality Reporting System) reporting, and other coding requirements. All of these have some stage of initial incentives that eventually turn to penalties or become required reporting.

In a little more than 10 years the United States has gone from paper charts, to electronic submissions, to electronic records. Under the rubric of simplification, privacy and security, and cost containment society is moving toward an increasingly standardized, if uncertain, electronic product.

EHRs have many strengths in terms of connectivity with hospitals and laboratories, e-prescriptions, and easy access to a patient's history and test results. However, there is a dark side to this technology that has a corrosive effect on quality. The expansion of the medical record into the electronic milieu has caused the concomitant growth of new problems. This article explores the issues of cloning in the medical record, auditing the EHR, and quality and quality programs.

CLONING IN THE MEDICAL RECORD

The term "cloning" is now being used quite openly by Medicare carriers and Medicare Administrative Contractors (MACs). Some federal documents use the term "repetitive documentation," some say cloning, but it is common knowledge what this means and how this plays out in professional practice.

In the early 2000s, the first electronic versions of office notes and progress records began to proliferate, and those early versions gave a first glimpse of the somewhat overlarge, disproportionate history and physical examination (PE) areas that have come to characterize many electronic notes. Although there had been dictation macros and printed templates in use for years that produced similar results, the electronic version of these seemed much more obvious if not actually different in content: they looked cloned.

Volume of Documentation Versus Medical Necessity

By 2004, Medicare produced guidance as to volume of documentation versus medical necessity. The Social Security Act, Section 1862 (a)(1)(A) states: "No payment will be made ... for items or services ...not reasonable and necessary for the diagnosis or treatment of an injury or illness or to improve the functioning of a malformed body member." This medical reasonableness and necessity standard is the overarching criterion for the payment for all services billed to Medicare. Providers frequently over-document and consequently select and bill for a higher-level E/M code than medically reasonable and necessary. Word processing software, the electronic medical record, and formatted note systems facilitate the "carry over" and repetitive "fill in" of stored information. Even if a complete note is generated, only the medically reasonable and necessary services for the condition of the particular patient at the time of the encounter as documented can be considered when selecting the appropriate level of an E/M service. Information that has no pertinence to the patient's situation at that specific time cannot be counted.[1]

When some practices purchase their EHR one of the selling points to the physician is that in the physician charting section every note could be constructed such that it opened up with, or started with, a complete normal review of systems (ROS) area and a complete normal PE. The rumble is that physicians and their practices may well be at risk depending on how much they rely on the preformatted version of ROS and PE that the EHR sets forth as a template. It has been clearly stated by Medicare carriers that overtemplating constitutes a medical necessity violation.

Cloning of Medical Notes

Documentation is considered cloned when each entry in the medical record for a beneficiary is worded exactly like or similar to the previous entries. Cloning also occurs when medical documentation is exactly the same from beneficiary to beneficiary. It would not be expected that every patient had the exact same problem and symptoms, and required the exact same treatment. Cloned documentation does not meet medical necessity requirements for coverage of services rendered because of the lack of specific, individual information. All documentation in the medical record must be specific to the patient and her or his situation at the time of the encounter. Cloning of documentation is considered a misrepresentation of the medical necessity requirement for coverage of services. Identification of this type of documentation leads to denial of services for lack of medical necessity and recoupment of all overpayments made.

Whether it is with EHR or transcription many providers use the same verbiage again and again in part to ensure they do not omit important information, in part because it is a habit. Any formatted documentation system can make things look repetitive, and there are aspects of the ROS and PE that are repetitive across most patients. Each provider usually finds their own voice and dictates, documents, and templates descriptive findings in their own way. This is normal and expected.

Thus, there are similarities and even identical things from visit to visit and across patients. That is why it is important to personalize these areas to each encounter. If the History of Present Illness (HPI) and Assessment/Plan (A/P) areas are well done they make that day's concerns and management apparent, but one does need to keep examinations and ROS in proportion to the event. Templates or

EHRs should be used judiciously and should include subjective information each time. It is the specificity of findings and management that must shine through the note, not the wallpaper.

Potentially Inappropriate Payments for Evaluation and Management Services

There is nothing ambiguous about the Federal statements regarding medical necessity. In 2012 the Health and Human Services Office of the Inspector General annual work plan included the following item: potentially inappropriate payments for evaluation and management services. Medicare contractors have noted an increased frequency of medical records with identical documentation across services: "We will also review multiple E&M services for the same providers and beneficiaries to identify electronic health records (EHR) documentation practices associated with potentially improper payments."[2]

As regulators see more and more notes that seem to have been written essentially by the machine, and are either out of proportion to or out of touch with the nature of the problems described in the HPI and A/P, they get the sense that the disjointed portions of the note may just be buffed or filler and designed to simply qualify for a higher level of service code. This would drive the costs of E/M services higher and do nothing to bend the cost curve. In fact, another 2012 Office of the Inspector General Work plan item addresses this directly, as discussed next.

Trends in Coding of Claims

We will review (E/M) claims to identify trends in the coding from 2000–2009. We will also identify providers that exhibited questionable billing for E/M services in 2009. Medicare paid $32 billion for E/M services in 2009, representing 19% of all Medicare Part B payments. Providers are responsible for ensuring that the codes they submit accurately reflect the services they provide.[3]

The trend that is of concern is a steady increase in the number of 99,214 Current Procedural Terminology code (level 4 established office visit) claims from year to year. Part of this is no doubt the concern that increased physician billings is in part supported by documentation that may not support medical necessity. The notion that EHRs are documenting, coding, and billing with minimal physician input is a real concern. It may seem like science fiction, but some systems can do all of that and the notion of these machine-generated notes uncoupled from actual physician work is a frightening prospect to regulatory and fiscal managers.

The truth is probably somewhere in between deliberate overcoding and overdocumentation, unconscious overdocumentation, and plain old user error. If there is too much of the same cookie-cutter portion of the record in the ROS and PE then likely the provider is just moving too quickly through these areas and not taking the time to customize findings. Some of this may just be careless, some may be the result of a cumbersome system, and it may just be haste. After all, the EHR just does what it is programmed to do.

However, there are errors that are just becoming too common. More disturbingly, there is an acceptance of this, an apathetic position that undermines quality of any sort.

Specific Quality Problems

The history
The Chief Complaint (CC) is where a patient history begins. Is a "here for follow-up" a CC? Is "here for labs" or "here for refills" a CC? How about "3-month visit" or some variation? Be specific; recent federal reviews have reported that there is

a lack of specific CCs. This is also the first documented section of the history; there-fore, one should make it count.

After the CC is the HPI. It is particularly disturbing to reviewers or auditors when elements of the HPI are contradicted in the ROS. The credibility of the whole note comes into question. Most likely this is a ROS that has been checked or clicked without being carefully reviewed and amended, but that is a quality issue. The real information is probably in the HPI, but which information in the note is real?

In documentation reviews the provider response to having these contradictions pointed out is often, "Oh yeah, I must have forgotten to correct that," or "the EHR was acting up that day," or even "I don't know how that got there." These records are signed off by the billing provider and sent out as a claim for payment. As such, the billing provider is the responsible party for the content of the note.

There complete Past, Family and Social Histories on problem-focused presenta-tions because the documentation system is most likely set to default to this all inclu-sive documentation. Although it is likely that some providers are quite attentive when it comes to keeping notes in proportion, it is just as likely many providers are not thinking about the proportion of their note, and click and send the document for payment. In the past, there was little or no discussion about proportion when notes were handwritten.

Medicare and specific MACs and carriers stake out their position on EHR documen-tation issues; however, there has not been a great deal of actual enforcement other than at the claims review level. As the number of EHR-users increases, the problem-prone areas will become more pervasive, and so too will the remedies.

The examination

When the CC or HPI are all about a particular body area or specific problem, but the documented examination for that area or system is identical to the last five patients who did not have issues in that area, there is another problem: the issue is introduced, but not addressed in the examination.

Medical Necessity of E/M services is based in part on the number, acuity and severity, and duration of problems addressed through history, PE, and medical decision-making. When documented clearly, the history, PE, and extent of medical decision-making associated with each problem is evident.

This latter issue is specifically proscribed in the Federal Documentation Guidelines. There it says, "A notation of normal or negative is sufficient for unaffected organ systems or body areas."[4] The idea being that for the areas involving the CC or present-ing problem that there be a specific narrative. Frequently the documentation is the usual canned examination of that organ system without the specificity suggested.

In the PE area one frequently sees "insight and judgment normal" as a neurologic or even psychiatric element. Does this documentation apply to a 4 year old? How about NCAT (Normo-Cephalic Atraumatic)? How often is this stated when it has no relevance to anything? It is often just an old habit. It is understood that some providers take the position that examinations are overrated to begin with, but one would not know it based on the volume of documentation produced in this area.

It is not uncommon to see providers document a minimum of eight organ systems on examination for every patient regardless of the nature of the complaint or problem. Even if they are not coding to the level of the examination, the relentless volume and bulk of these documentation elements detract from the focus of the encounter and contribute to the sense of bloated notes.

Clinicians are all familiar with the story of the patient who comes back from the consulting physician's office, and has the consultant note describing a comprehensive history and examination. Then the patient says that "I never took my clothes off" or they were "only in the room for 2 minutes." This is fraud. Where is the quality there?

Medical Decision-Making or Assessment and Plan

Medical decision-making or the Assessment and Plan section of the medical note has always been the most important part of the paper or electronic chart. The history and examination are the methods and means that providers use to gather data. Most medical necessity determinations hinge on this element and this is where the provider must make clear the problems, the status of the problems, and the treatment and the management of the problems. EHRs have helped and hindered in this regard, and are influenced by the system and software purchased and the user of such.

Part of the issue is that the medical record now has many users: the clinician, the insurance company, the regulators, and researchers. What communicates clearly among physicians does not necessarily communicate to the others. One of the biggest issues is how different EHRs format the A/P. In many cases, a list is generated and nothing more.

The Assessment section of the medical record is often followed by the Plan. Although the Plan area may outline treatments, it may not clearly link them to the problems in the Assessment. This is a problem on the regulatory side. What about those problems listed in the plan that have no or seem to have no corresponding treatment or management in the plan? Are these being managed today? Are they comorbidities that pertain to today's problems? Are they simply historical elements? Is the provider using the Assessment area as a running problem list?

All of these versions can be true but all leave it unclear in the mind of the reviewer what was actually managed on the date of service. Again, conventions here can hurt in a Medical Necessity review. Perhaps the biggest shortfall of most systems is the lack of ability to characterize the problems easily in the Assessment area.

The decision-making element of E/M codes is based in large part on the status of a given problem (ie, is it stable, worsening, or severely exacerbated). The list of problems most often does not include the status. Often it can be inferred from the management below, but this leaves the determination to the knowledge and intuition of the reviewer, not always good for the provider. Perhaps the most important effort a provider can make in this area is to be certain that the number and status of each problem is clear.

The 1997 Federal Documentation Guidelines state that:

For a presenting problem with an established diagnosis the record should reflect whether the problem is:

a. Improved, well controlled, resolving or resolved; or,
b. Inadequately controlled, worsening, or failing to change as expected.

For a presenting problem without an established diagnosis, the assessment or clinical impression may be stated in the form of differential diagnoses or as a 'possible,' 'probable,' or 'rule out' diagnosis.[5]

Getting here often involves typing and more keystrokes in a text area under the Assessment or the Plan section of the note, so the course of least resistance is to let the list stand, without characterization. It is somewhat insidious that the most important keystrokes come last in the note, when one has already navigated numerous screens, menus, and pathways.

Preprogrammed management options, such as "continue same medications" and "refill all," have long been discouraged by federal payers as not specific enough because one would not know which medications for which problems. This leads reviewers back to comparing lists, not the specificity for which they are looking.

Many systems allow one to create specific management macros or paragraphs to address common issues. However, this too can get out of hand. Let us say that a patient is scheduled for a chronic disease follow-up visit to address four of five problems. The provider deals with them, then starts clicking the management macros that go with each problem in addition to the medication updates or changes. The result is five paragraphs going into great depth about the five different diets that were discussed and all the handouts that were gone over in detail. This brings us back to the cloned appearance of things because it looks like too much information. The intent was good, the execution somewhat overdone. Appearances count here and so does the patient's recollection of the experience.

Another area of concern is documentation of time spent counseling or coordinating care. One EHR allows the providers to code an encounter based solely on time, and offers the provider a place to enter the total encounter time. But the text it generates and appends at the end of the note says, "Over half of 'x' time spent counseling and/or coordinating care." These words are not only generic in fact and appearance, but are not even a statement. The effective way to document time is to integrate a statement about time spent into the narrative in the A/P.

AUDITING THE EHR

The documentation issues outlined previously involve proportion, contradictory statements, and lists of things that are either unclear or just look contrived among others. Some of these are obvious when looking at a single note, whereas others become more visible in aggregate, then patterns emerge.

One would think that one element of documentation that the EHR addressed was the identity of the provider. After all, there are now electronic signatures and security protocols to handle this. Well, maybe not. One of the largest systems on the market, frequently found in large teaching environments, has the resident signature at the top of the page, before the note. When the rest of the note unfolds, and then the attending provides either an attestation or some corroboratory findings, there is no signature to mark where one leaves off and the other begins. True, there is usually a way to look at keystrokes and log-ins on most systems, but this is more of a forensic approach and the note itself does not make it clear who did what.

The attestations themselves, required in some fashion for resident/attending notes since 1969 have now become formulaic and were perhaps the original chart element to go macro. CMS Transmittal 811 states:

When using an electronic medical record, it is acceptable for the teaching physician to use a macro as the required personal documentation if the teaching physician adds it personally in a secured (password protected) system.

In addition to the teaching physician's macro, either the resident or the teaching physician must provide customized information that is sufficient to support a medical necessity determination.

The note in the electronic medical record must sufficiently describe the specific services furnished to the specific patient on the specific date. It is insufficient documentation if the resident and the teaching physician use macros only.[6]

A careful read of this last sentence indicates that as long both attending and resident do not use macros (presumably for the entirety of the note), then it is acceptable if one does. What happens is the attending faculty uses generic macros on top of the resident detail.

This is not really what CMS had in mind when they created the attending participation guidelines. There is typically great variance among attending faculty within a given academic setting relating to the extent to which they demonstrate participation. Some use macros alone, some add a brief note, some write full notes every time. Between the cloned ROS, PE, and managements macros in the resident note, and often the all macro-attending note, CMS is paying new money every-time for some well-used parts. Almost half of some notes are recognizably cookie-cutter. Again, the question arises: is this quality, efficiency, or expediency.

Note the emphasis in Transmittal 811 on subjective information. The word "customized" speaks directly to the overuse of generic information. CMS is signaling that they are watching carefully the use of cloned notes.

Finally, the coup de gras of the EHR for training institutions, statements above the attestations that say "the above note reflects the combined work of the resident and the attending. The note has been edited and amended by me, the attending, and includes my corrections." This is interesting for two reasons: one can really no longer tell which work belongs to whom and thus cannot audit it, and this amendment and semi-attestation has itself become more of a macro than anything, totally generic, including the identification of the attending. This alone is insufficient as an attestation and does not meet Federal criteria. It is also an example of how technology and modern usage has outstripped the ability of the regulations to monitor them. The teaching guidelines, updated in November 2011, were written to deal with two distinct notes in relation to one another, not a blended note.

Beyond note attribution and attestation, what about content? How does one audit things like the following:

- No CC (the guidelines state that there must be one, and that it can be part of the HPI. There is no mention of mutual exclusivity)
- (HPI) no complaints
- (ROS) ROS negative
- (ROS) ROS per the HPI (but there is no ROS in the HPI)
- ROS otherwise negative except as specifically noted in the HPI (no ROS in the HPI)
- Complete 14, system review performed and negative except as mentioned in the HPI (as above)
- Examination unremarkable
- Examination unchanged since last visit
- (A/P), Follow-up in 6 weeks
- Continue same
- RTC (return to clinic) as needed

Medicare does not think much of these practices and would not recognize them on review if used as often seen. Some are specifically disallowed. But are the more polished and detailed appearing version of these any more acceptable, such as the ROS that provides great detail on each of the 14 systems every time? What about the documented examination that covers every organ system and body area, in detail, every time? When does the auditor say, "I just don't believe that you did all that for this problem"?

Remember the line, "Information that has no pertinence to the patient's situation at that specific time cannot be counted."[7] Overdocumentation is about to be as much of a problem as underdocumentation. Keep in mind that MACs and carriers are required to perform probe audits to validate correctly paid claims. With $32-plus billion in annual payments for E/M codes from Medicare alone, one can bet that any sense of a runaway train here will be monitored.

QUALITY AND QUALITY PROGRAMS

Accountable care organizations and programs designed to improve value, increase quality, and cut costs, such as the Patient Centered Medical Home, are laudable in scope and vision but some of the execution has fallen short in the deployment, oversight, and management of health information technology. In the same way that we have hopefully demonstrated that EHRs are very good at keeping a record of what it says someone did, the fear here is that we will soon have a great track record of quality measures that we say we did.

Already the CMS Physician Quality Reporting System is paying bonuses on Category II Current Procedural Terminology code reporting that is now generated by the EHR. Some of the measures call for actual measurements that are recorded and that is somewhat tangible, but some call for counseling and other intangibles.

Besides the obvious quality benefit to the patient if the actual elements of the program are performed, many networks are vying for patient-centered medical home certification because of the anticipated increased payments it will yield. The requirements of some of these programs are daunting: follow-up on every laboratory test, every referral, and prescription; a requirement that the follow-up be documented; or maybe just that a box be checked.

Who is doing all of this follow-up, and scanning referrals, faxes, and forms into the e-chart? Is that cost effective? Are all the extra touches really contributing to quality of care, or is it just more busy work, more energy toward a perfect chart that says one did everything one was supposed to do and more?

HOW DID WE GET HERE?

In 1995 and 1997, Medicare published its Federal Documentation Guidelines. These guidelines provided the documentation rules associated with each code. As above, in the 1990s and throughout the last decade came the push for electronic claims and EHRs.

Are the EHR issues described just the adolescence of the electronic era or indicative or suggestive of a pervasive lack of quality, a willingness to let these frequently corrupted notes stand? There are so many reasons offered for why notes are as bad as they frequently are, mostly about time, or an unfriendly or dysfunctional system. There are tremendous downward pressures on physicians to interface and multitask as never before. At the end of the day it seems to come down to operator error as often as not.

This article does not touch on the ethics, or real fraud, or the lesser degrees of fraud committed every day, the latter sometimes unknowingly. Moreover, it also does not touch on the stress and frustration experienced by all members of the health care team when implementing an EHR. Systems that provide ongoing training and real-time assistance to clinicians and others working to provide care, treatment, and services to patients and be paid for the work they are doing requires proactive leadership. At the end of the day (preferably at the end of each visit), providers need to document their interaction in the form of a real note to reflect the specific care provided to a patient on the date of service.

REFERENCES

1. The Social Security Act, Section 1862 (a)(1)(A). Available at: www.ssa.gov/OP_Home/ssact/title18/1862.htm.

2. Part 1: Medicare Part A, Part B, p. 20 "Potentially inappropriate payments for evaluation and management services." Available at: http://oig.hhs.gov/reports-and-publications/archives/workplan/2012/Work-Plan-2012.pdf.

3. Part 1: Medicare Part A, Part B, p. 19. "Trends in coding of claims." Available at: http://oig.hhs.gov/reports-and-publications/archives/workplan/2012/Work-Plan-2012.pdf.

4. Documentation Guidelines for Evaluation and Management (E/M...2012). 1997 Documentation Guidelines for Evaluation and Management Services. "A notation of normal or negative is sufficient for unaffected organ systems or body areas." Available at: www.cms.gov/Outreach-and-Education/Medicare./EMDOC.html.

5. Documentation Guidelines for Evaluation and Management (E/M..2012). 1997 Documentation Guidelines for Evaluation and Management Services. Available at: www.cms.gov/Outreach-and-Education/Medicare./EMDOC.html.

6. CMS Transmittal 811 states: "It is insufficient documentation if the resident and the teaching physician use macros only." Available at: https://www.cms.gov/Outreach-and-Education/Outreach/PRIT/Past-PRIT-Issues-Items/CMS062947.html.

7. "Information that has no pertinence to the patient's situation at that specific time cannot be counted." Available at: http://www.flmedical.org/Index.aspx.

Utilizing International Medical Graduates in Health Care Delivery
Brain Drain, Brain Gain, or Brain Waste? A Win-Win Approach at University of California, Los Angeles

Patrick T. Dowling, MD, MPH[a],*, Michelle Anne Bholat, MD, MPH[b]

KEYWORDS

- Affordable Care Act • Brain drain • Brain waste • International medical graduates
- Medical migration • Health disparities • Limited english proficiency
- Linguistic barriers to care

KEY POINTS

- At present, 25% of America's physician workforce is represented by international medical graduates (IMGs).
- Few IMGs are from Latin America, even although America's Hispanic population now exceeds 50 million, represented by 18 million foreign-born or 36% of the Hispanic population. In California, Hispanics represent 37% of the population, yet only 5.5% of the physician workforce. After identifying a large number of unlicensed Hispanic IMGs legally residing in southern California, the University of California, Los Angeles (UCLA) developed an innovative program to prepare these sidelined physicians, who were often working in menial jobs, to enter family medicine residency programs in the state and become licensed physicians with the skills necessary to provide cost-effective, high-quality health care.
- On completion of a 3-year California family medicine residency-training program, these IMGs have an obligation to practice in a federally designated underserved community in the state for 2 to 3 years.
- As the US health care system continues the journey of transformation from physician-centered practices to patient-focused teams, with primary care serving as the foundation for building patient-centered medical homes to neighborhoods, attention to educating IMGs in these concepts is crucial, given that this group represents 25% of the US physician workforce.

[a] Department of Family Medicine, Geffen School of Medicine at UCLA, Box 951683, Los Angeles, CA 90095, USA; [b] Department of Family Medicine, UCLA Family Health Center, Geffen School of Medicine at UCLA, 1920 Colorado Avenue, Santa Monica, CA 90404, USA
* Corresponding author.
E-mail address: pdowling@mednet.ucla.edu

Prim Care Clin Office Pract 39 (2012) 643–648
http://dx.doi.org/10.1016/j.pop.2012.08.002
0095-4543/12/$ – see front matter © 2012 Elsevier Inc. All rights reserved.

INTRODUCTION

Although not a new phenomenon, the transnational migration of individuals has increased over the past several years as the rapid pace of globalization has opened borders to not only goods and services but millions of workers as well. There are now more than 215 million individuals, or 3.1% of the world's population of 7 billion, living outside their country of birth.[1,2] Although often overlooked amid the current controversies over the influx of poor undocumented immigrants in the United States, legal immigration has resulted in a significant number of well-educated immigrants, including health professionals.[3]

Immigration Law Changes and the Passage of Medicare and Medicaid

In the early 1960s, the Kennedy administration liberalized immigration policy by replacing a 40-year-old national quota system, which favored immigrants from Northern Europe, with a more flexible policy that favored immigrants from the eastern hemisphere. Further, it gave preference to highly skilled and educated immigrants who could alleviate personal shortages in the nation.[4]

With the passage of Medicare and Medicaid legislation in 1965, millions of seniors and low-income Americans were provided with health insurance, resulting in an increased demand for health care. However, access remained problematic because of an existing physician shortage. Soon thereafter, many physicians began immigrating to the United States seeking hospital-based graduate medical education (GME) training positions. Most of these international medical graduates (IMGs) originated from resource-poor counties in the southern hemisphere and immigrated to the wealthy countries of the northern hemisphere.[3,5]

Impact of Medical Migration

Countries of origin

Although most immigrated with the intent to return to their home country after obtaining specialty training, this situation changed over time, because only 10% returned home permanently. As a result, IMGs in America now number 210,000 and account for 25% of America's physician workforce.[5,6]

After half a century, the migration of physicians from resource-poor counties to developed countries has resulted in immense imbalances in the global health workforce and what many view as a brain drain.[5–7] Although these countries were already faced with an inadequate infrastructure because of a shortage of well-trained health workers, the further loss perpetuates and exacerbates a preexisting maldistribution of health and financial resources away from those populations most in need of basic health services. Consequently, those countries with the highest burden of diseases now have the fewest number of health workers, whereas those with significantly lower disease burdens have the largest health care workforce.

The greatest disparity exists in the Sub-Saharan region of Africa, which has 25% of the world's disease burden, yet only 3% of the world's health workers and 1% of the world's economic resources to meet the challenge.[6] Moreover, this loss of health professionals is occurring in the face of a ravaging epidemic of chronic infectious diseases: human immunodeficiency virus/AIDS, malaria, and tuberculosis, and a growing epidemic of chronic noncommunicable diseases, such as heart disease and diabetes, particularly among the urban poor.[6–8]

Further, many view this emigration or fatal flow of skilled health care workers from Africa as paramount to a silent theft of public funds that poor countries had earmarked to subsidize medical education by developed countries, including the United States, that fail to fund and create sufficient educational capacity consonant with their own national needs.[4,6,9]

Although many have lamented this drain of educated health professionals, no substantive actions had been taken until government leaders from several African nations began publicizing that some host countries were poaching their health professionals, because the evidence suggested active recruiting in Africa for health care workers. After a decade of discussion, the World Health Organization successfully brokered the adoption of a code of practice on international recruitment of health professionals.[10,11]

Brain Drain or Brain Waste in America

Although America relies on IMGs to meet its unmet needs, only a few IMGs from Africa have immigrated here. As a result of pull factors (opportunities, political stability, physician earnings) combined with push factors in source countries, America remains a magnet for graduate medical training from IMG applicants worldwide. Last year, more than 11,107 IMGs applied for, and 4877 were accepted into, a first-year GME position in the United States.[10,12] There is no active recruiting in Africa or any other country.

A different issue with respect to medical migration exists in America, namely brain waste, a term that is used to describe 1.3 million skilled immigrants in America with a college degree or higher who are currently working below their skill levels, often in menial jobs.[12-14] A World Bank study found striking differences in the occupational level attained by immigrants with similar educational backgrounds by country. Controlling for all variables, the research showed that highly educated immigrants from several Latin American, Eastern European, and Middle Eastern countries had a low likelihood of obtaining skilled jobs here compared with those from Asia and Western Europe. Further, they found that a large part of this country-level variation could be explained by certain country attributes, such as expenditure on tertiary education and the use of English as a medium of education.[14]

According to Batalova and Fix,[13] brain waste has consequences for immigrants, because it means bringing home less money than they have the potential to earn, as well as for the country overall, because it represents a missed opportunity to leverage already trained professionals in areas where there may be a desperate need for them.

Immigrant Doctors and Immigrant Patients in America: Brain Gain or Brain Waste?

There are now 38 million immigrants in the United States, 47% of whom are from Latin American and 25% from Asia. Overall, the Hispanic population now exceeds 50 million, whereas the Asian population has grown to 18 million.[15] Given the considerable number of these 2 minority populations and their respective immigrant subpopulations, a logical question is to ask what percentage from each group is represented by the 210,000 IMGs living in the United States.

A study on the country of citizenship of foreign IMGs in America, at the time of medical school entry, documented that not one of the top 10 countries of origin of immigrant IMGs is a Latin American nation, whereas the 3 top source countries are represented by immigrants from India, Pakistan, and the Philippines.[16]

Linguistic Barriers and Health Care Disparities in California

Almost 30% of America's Hispanic population (nearly 15 million) reside in California and represent 37% of the state's 38 million people, yet account for 59% of the state's 7 million uninsured. Further, California Hispanics have the highest uninsured rate, the highest poverty rate, and the lowest educational attainment compared with any population in the state. Each of these population characteristics represents barriers to health care access. Collectively, they coalesce into a multidimensional barrier, and as a result, Hispanics are disproportionately at risk for not having access to basic care.[17]

Complicating barriers to health care access is limited English proficiency (LEP). Nearly two-thirds of the state's 6.9 million people with LEP are Hispanic, and those individuals with both LEP and lack of insurance (the so-called double burden) confront the greatest barriers to care. A survey found that two-thirds of uninsured Spanish-speaking Hispanics did not have a usual source of care (USOC) compared with 37% of non-Hispanic whites, 44% of Blacks, and 46% of English-speaking Hispanics. Having a USOC is crucial, because it can blunt some of the effects of being uninsured by providing a direct conduit to access when needed.[18]

The Institute of Medicine has documented that a diverse physician workforce results in fewer medical errors, better outcomes, and higher patient satisfaction if the workforce mirrors, to some degree, the population being served.[19] The diversity of the physician workforce has not been achieved in California, because Hispanics represent just 5.5% of the state's physician workforce.[20]

The Affordable Care Act, Health Disparities, and the Patient-Centered Medical Home

The passage of the Affordable Care Act means that up to 32 million currently uninsured Americans will gain insurance, 4.5 million of whom are in California. Although more than 2 million Hispanics will gain health insurance in California, many will not be able to access quality health care because of nonfinancial barriers related to language and culture. In an attempt to address the substantial gaps in the US health care system between current practices and optimal care, the patient-centered medical home (PCMH) has emerged as a centerpiece of efforts to reform health care delivery and to establish a primary care basis for improving the efficacy of health care. Rather than advocating for a narrow approach to organize health care, the PCMH seeks to personalize, prioritize, and integrate care to improve the health of individuals and populations. It is based on the fundamental tenets of primary care: access, comprehensiveness, coordination, and a continuity relationship with a personal physician.[21]

Like much of the nation, California lacks a primary care workforce that is adequate in size and diversity to address the nonfinancial barriers necessary to ensure effective access for many. Given its large monolingual Hispanic immigrant population, its primary care workforce needs to be diverse enough to address the cultural and linguistic barriers to effective care that thousands of these newly insured individuals encounter. Given that the gap between the size of California's Hispanic population compared with the number of health professionals able to effectively communicate is widening, we elected to confront the demographic reality of California by developing a an innovative approach to improve care for these monolingual Hispanic patients through a resourceful approach that increases the supply of bicultural, bilingual Hispanic family physicians in California.

An Innovative Program Linking Hispanic IMGs to Improving Community Health

The University of California, Los Angeles (UCLA) Department of Family Medicine developed a novel program to increase the number of bilingual, bicultural Hispanic family physicians in the state, drawing on the pool of those sidelined physicians who had emigrated from Latin America but were working at or near minimum wage. Although many were working in health care, they were in positions significantly below their level of education, whereas others worked as food handlers, factory workers, custodians, and in other low-paying jobs. With more than 1400 applications and hundreds of interviews, these IMGs reported that they immigrated to America with the dream of obtaining a medical license and practicing medicine. In their spare time many were preparing for the 3 US medical licensing examinations (USMLEs) required to gain entrance into a residency training program, a prerequisite for medical licensure in California. Overwhelmingly, they lacked in-depth knowledge of the testing process, and the best methods to prepare. Moreover, few understood the competitive nature of the process and the fact that English skills were crucial to obtaining high scores.

In 2006, a unique and comprehensive preresidency training program was developed with approval from the Dean of the David School of Medicine at UCLA to address the diversity of the physician workforce to meet the needs of California's Hispanic communities. Initially, the curriculum focused on how to best prepare these IMGs to successfully pass the USMLE examinations and improve professional-level English oral and writing skills. The curriculum was developed to help UCLA IMGs to successfully prepare an application to a California family medicine residency training program and provide a clinical observership for IMGs to learn the language and culture of US medicine. In 2009, the observership increased from 8 weeks to 12 weeks, and in 2010, the outpatient curriculum expanded to include the core concepts of the PCMH. The Institute for Healthcare Improvement (IHI) Open School PCMH curriculum, which is required as part of the clinical training and plans to institute IHI's population health, will be added to the curriculum in 2013 to give the UCLA IMGs the basic tools to work effectively in other settings that have adopted the PCMH model of care.

The UCLA IMG program is free of tuition or fees, covers all educational expenses, and includes a small stipend. In return, the IMGs must agree to apply only to family medicine training programs in California and to practice in an underserved community in the state for 2 to 3 years after completion of training. Because this is a full-time program, the length of enrollment ranges from 4 to 21 and is supported entirely by private funding.

Since its inception in 2006, the program has placed 54 program graduates into family medicine residency programs, including 13 graduates in June 2012. All but 1 IMG completed a California program. In comparison, the 10 California medical schools graduate an average of 14 Hispanic graduates per year, most of who do not choose careers in family medicine.

Consistent with recommendations of the Institute of Medicine's *Crossing the Quality Chasm* report,[1] the UCLA IMG program represents the patient-centeredness that is a necessary core component of a health care system designed to improve the quality of care.[22] It mirrors the PCMH concept that a personal physician is needed to assess patient needs, based on their family, cultural, and linguistic background, as well as their health, lifestyle, and health care literacy to improve and create better outcomes.

Furthermore, this program successfully addresses a likely brain waste by providing these unlicensed IMGs with the tools to compete for the GME needed for licensure to practice. The result is a group of residency-trained board-certified family physicians who can address the linguistic and cultural barriers to care (key to the PCMH) for the same immigrant population from Latin American countries from whence they have come. Not to do so would represent a missed opportunity to leverage already trained professionals in areas where there is a desperate need for them as well as being a waste of education and talent.

REFERENCES

1. United Nations Department of Economic and Social Affairs Population Division. Trends in International Migrant Stock: The 2008 Revision. 2009. Available at: http://esa.un.org/migration/index.asp?panel=1. Accessed July 3, 2012.
2. International Organization on Migration, About migration, facts and figures. Available at: http://www.iom.int/jahia/Jahia/about-migration/facts-and-figures/lang/en. Accessed July 8, 2012.

3. Gureje O, Hollins S. Report of WPA task force on brain drain. World Psychiatry 2009;8(2):115–8.
4. Irigoyen M, Zambrana R. Foreign medical graduates (FMGs): determining their role in the U.S. health care system. Soc Sci Med 1979;13A:775–83.
5. Mullan F. The metrics of the physician brain drain. N Engl J Med 2005;353:1810–8.
6. Chen L, Boufford JI. Fatal flows–doctors on the move. N Engl J Med 2005;335:1850–2.
7. Mayosi BM, Flisher AJ, Lalloo UG, et al. The burden of non-communicable diseases in South Africa. Lancet 2009;374:934–47.
8. Daar AS, Singer PA, Persad DL, et al. Grand challenges in chronic non-communicable diseases. Nature 2007;450:494–5.
9. Hussey PS. International migration patterns of physicians to the U.S. Health Policy 2007;84:298–307.
10. Taylor AL, Hwenda L, Larsen B. Stemming the brain drain–a WHO global cost of practice on international recruitment of health personnel. N Engl J Med 2011;365:2348–50.
11. Sheikh M. Commitment and action to boost health workforce. Lancet 2012;379:e2–3.
12. National Resident Matching Program, Results and Data: 2012 Main Residency. Available at: http://www.nrmp.org/data. Accessed June 18, 2012.
13. Batalova J, Fix M. Uneven progress: the employment pathways of skilled immigrants in the United States. Washington, DC: Migration Policy Institute; 2008. Available at: http://www.migrationpolicy.org/pubs/BrainWasteOct08.pdf. Accessed June 15, 2012.
14. Mattoo A, Ozden C, Neaqu C. Brain waste? Educated immigrants in the U.S. labor market. World Bank policy research working paper no. 3581: World Bank Development Research Group (DECRG). World Bank; 2005.
15. Patten E. Statistical portrait of the foreign-born population in the United States. 2010. Available at: http://www.pewhispanic.org/. Accessed July 7, 2012.
16. Boulet JR, Norcini JJ, Whelan GP. The international medical graduate pipeline: recent trends in certification and residency training. Health Aff 2006;25(2):469–77.
17. Kaiser Family Foundation. State health facts. California, demographics and the economy. Available at: http://www.statehealthfacts.org/profileglance.jsp?rgn=6&;rgn=1&showall=1. Accessed July 3, 2012.
18. Doty MM. Hispanic patients' double burden: lack of health insurance and limited English. The Commonwealth Fund. 2003. Available at: http://www.commonwealthfund.org/Publications/Fund-Reports/2003/. Accessed July 1, 2012.
19. Smedley BD, Bulter AS, Breslow LR. In the nation's compelling interest: ensuring diversity in the health-care workforce. Committee on Institutional and Policy-level Strategies for Increasing the Diversity of the U.S. Healthcare. National Academies Press; 2004.
20. AMA physician profile, American Medical Association, Division of Survey and Data Resources. Chicago (IL): American Medical Association; 2011.
21. Strange KC, Nutting PA, Miller WL, et al. Defining and measuring the patient-centered medical home. J Gen Intern Med 2010;25:601–12.
22. Institute of Medicine. Crossing the quality chasm: a new health system for the 21st century. Committee on Quality of Health Care. Washington, DC: National Academies Press; 2001.

Adoption of Self-Management Interventions for Prevention and Care

Mary Jane Rotheram-Borus, PhD[a],*, Barbara L. Ingram, PhD[b],
Dallas Swendeman, PhD[a], Adabel Lee, PhD[a]

KEYWORDS

- Self-management • Self-regulation • Chronic illness • Chronic disease
- Interventions • Prevention

KEY POINTS

- Self-management interventions (SMI) improve health-related quality of life, reduce health care costs, and prevent progression of chronic conditions.
- Five elements of SMIs are activating motivation, applying information, developing skills, acquiring environmental resources, and building social support.
- These elements are as relevant to disease prevention in healthy people as they are to management of chronic diseases.
- Development of self-management competence is conceptualized in three phases (motivate, action, maintenance); interventions must be tailored to the phase.
- Delivery vehicles for SMIs range from traditional primary care settings to use of technological innovations.

Health care costs in the United States are reaching unprecedented heights. In 2009, health care spending was $2.5 trillion, $8086 per person, or 17.6% of the gross domestic product (GDP),[1] making it the second highest in the world. Despite this huge financial investment, the life expectancy of people in the United States ranks last on a list of 11 wealthy nations and ranks fiftieth in the world. The average life expectancy for American men is 76.05 years compared with 78.89 years for Canadian men.[2] In 2005, 43.8% of the US civilian, noninstitutionalized population had 1 or more chronic conditions.[3] The economic burden of chronic illness is currently 78% of total health care spending,[4] and 96% of Medicare annual spending is for chronic conditions.[5] It is estimated that by 2023, there will be a 42% increase in cases of 7 major chronic diseases, costing $4.2 trillion in treatment costs and lost economic output.[6]

[a] Global Center for Children and Families, Semel Institute for Neuroscience and Human Behavior, 10920 Wilshire Boulevard, Suite 350, University of California at Los Angeles, Los Angeles, CA 90024-6521, USA; [b] Graduate School of Education and Psychology, Pepperdine University, 6100 Center Drive, Los Angeles, CA 90045, USA
* Corresponding author.
E-mail address: rotheram@ucla.edu

Prim Care Clin Office Pract 39 (2012) 649–660
http://dx.doi.org/10.1016/j.pop.2012.08.006
0095-4543/12/$ – see front matter © 2012 Published by Elsevier Inc.
primarycare.theclinics.com

Lifestyle change is the key to reducing the human and financial burden of chronic disease by preventing disease and delaying advancement of disease. Four risk factors directly contribute to the prevalence and severity of chronic illnesses, as well as their prevention: unhealthy diet, physical inactivity, tobacco use, and alcohol abuse.[7] These lifestyle factors—primarily determined by the individual and often not addressed by medical providers—were the leading cause of death in 2000, with tobacco causing 18.1% of deaths, poor diet and physical inactivity causing 16.1% of deaths, and alcohol consumption causing 3.5% of all deaths. The significance of patients' behavioral choices places patient self-management at the center of chronic care and prevention models.[8,9]

SELF-MANAGEMENT AS THE GOLD STANDARD OF CHRONIC CARE

The World Health Organization's (WHO) best practice strategy for chronic conditions is to "educate and support patients to manage their own conditions as much as possible."[10] The outcome of a self-management approach is a change in the physician–patient relationship. The patient becomes an active, informed, collaborative participant in health care decision-making; assumes responsibility for engaging in health-promoting behaviors and relationships; and develops competence for problem solving and proactively addressing predictable challenges of the disease.[8,11] Chronic illness self-management and healthy lifestyle promotion for the prevention of disease require similar cognitive processes to transform intentions into behavior: capacity for self-evaluation; self-managed action with task- and time-specific, outcome-focused goal setting[12]; active patient involvement; and ongoing planning.[13]

The outcome of self-management interventions (SMIs) is that patients have the skills to monitor markers of health and disease, make decisions to modify their own behavior, and develop individualized goal-setting and action plans. Chodosh and colleagues[14] defined self-management as having a minimum of two components—self-monitoring and decision-making. Creer and colleagues[11] described it as using "the capacity for self-evaluation and self-managed action." Furthermore, because chronic diseases often limit patients' aspirations (eg, diabetes may stop a rock climber from achieving his goals), patients must accept their losses, find new goals to engage in,[15] and develop competence in coping with failure, known as relapse management.[16]

Two comprehensive meta-analyses of SMI studies using randomized trials[14,17] found positive outcomes for patients with diabetes, hypertension, arthritis, and asthma. Three reviews that included studies with nonrandomized methodologies[18–20] reported benefits for patients with asthma, arthritis, diabetes, and hypertension. Multiple literature reviews, as well as primary source data, show consensus about a set of common factors for effective self-management.[11,21–24]

NECESSARY ELEMENTS FOR EFFECTIVE SELF-MANAGEMENT

The essential elements for successful self-management are organized within 5 categories: (1) activate motivation for change, (2) apply information from education and self-monitoring, (3) develop skills, (4) acquire environmental resources, and (5) build social support. These same elements can contribute to successful health maintenance of people who are currently healthy, and thus should be viewed as essential elements of prevention as well as chronic disease management.

Element 1: Activate Motivation for Change

Every SMI program includes educational components or intervention techniques (eg, motivational interviewing) to create motivation to engage in health-promoting behaviors, usually by enhancing individuals' beliefs in their ability to achieve desired change (self-efficacy). To be activated to change, the individual needs to accept responsibility for lifestyle change and experience a sense of empowerment,[25,26] counteracting feelings of being a victim of the illness by feeling in control of their disease. The patient needs to resolve intergoal conflict[27] and value health and longevity more than the gratifications of the current lifestyle, which may include the pleasures of enjoying rich food, alcohol, cigarettes, and sedentary forms of recreation. Cultural roles and beliefs must be recognized to motivate change. For example, women in many cultures are socialized to value the needs of family members above their own, and will not serve healthier meals (eg, reduced fat, smaller portions) to the whole family, unless they frame that choice as protection rather than deprivation. Motivation to change is likely to be stronger for disease management than for prevention.[13]

The stages of change model[28] applies to self-management commitment[29] and describes how an individual is more likely to change behavior when an intervention matches his or her stage of change. Participants in a self-management treatment for chronic pain were less likely to complete the program if they were judged to be in the precontemplation or contemplation stage, rather than the preparation or action stage.[30] Motivational interviewing,[31] a technique based on the stages of change model, has been used in health settings to move patients to commit to change.[32,33]

Maintenance of change over time needs to receive as much focus as initial behavior change.[34] Setbacks arise from unexpected declines in health despite adherence to health-promoting plans and need to be framed as challenges to overcome, rather than reasons to relapse to unhealthy behaviors. Cognitive interventions are helpful at this stage, as people are best prepared for setbacks when they have internalized thought patterns that protect against disengagement.[15]

Element 2: Apply Information

Education is an essential component of SMI. Patients need information about the disease as well as the general chronic care model. Another source of information is self-observation and self-recording on a regular, established schedule, enabling the patient to modify medication and behaviors without direct supervision of a health care professional.[11] Self-monitoring comprises of 2 processes: (1) awareness of bodily symptoms, sensations, daily activities, and cognitive processes and (2) measurements, recordings, and observations that provide information for independent action or consultation with care providers.[35] Self-management is enhanced when patients can gather information about the status of their physical health by monitoring specific markers of biologic functioning on a daily basis. For example, glycemic level monitored through blood testing is the marker for diabetes; blood pressure and heart rate are markers for cardiovascular conditions; and airflow is the marker for asthma and chronic obstructive pulmonary disease (COPD). Self-monitoring of psychological states such as depressed mood, anxiety, and fatigue is another essential component of self-regulation,[36] as psychological states can often impact physical health and adherence to medical regimens. The creation of methods for patients to monitor biomarkers of stress is an important future goal, especially for people living with human immunodeficiency virus (HIV).[37]

Element 3: Skill Development

Patients need skills to manage their specific disease, maintain health-promoting behaviors, and use behavior change technology for problem solving and creation of action plans. Effective communication and collaboration with health care providers are common outcome goals in health interventions and necessary skills for self-management.[18,23,38,39] Ideally, patients are empowered to manage their health and their disease through a partnership[8] in which patients and practitioners enter into collaborative problem solving and agree upon mutually negotiated goals.[40] Disease-specific skills include appropriate use of devices (eg, an inhaler for asthma or a blood pressure monitor for cardiovascular disease), adherence to complicated medication programs, and the ability to interpret new symptoms.[38] Generic health-related skills include those needed for initiating and maintaining lifestyle changes and dealing with psychological distress.[41] Specific skills for overcoming obstacles and challenges will vary depending on the individual person and his or her health status. Five of the most important skills are highlighted in the following sections.

Problem-solving

Frequently cited as the most important skill, problem solving is a prerequisite for successful self-management, and it can be viewed as a mediator of improved health outcomes.[13] Problem solving is typically described as a series of steps: identifying the problem, setting a goal, generating possible solutions, selecting and implementing an action plan, and readjusting plans until goals are reached. Information-seeking skills are part of every phase in problem solving.

Self-monitoring

Self-monitoring motivates and maintains behavior change by promoting self-efficacy, increasing awareness, and monitoring progress. Self-monitoring has been used effectively to change dietary behaviors through use of food-tracking instruments.[42]

Stress management and emotional regulation

Coping with negative emotions is a major task for people living with chronic illness.[43] Because depression is a condition that impedes successful self-management,[44,45] skills for preventing and managing dysphoric moods are extremely beneficial.

Coping with lapses and setbacks

To cope effectively with lapses, and prevent them from becoming excuses to revert to unhealthy behavior patterns, individuals must have cognitive strategies for framing their behavior as a predictable part of the learning curve, rather than failure.[46] For long-term lifestyle change, individuals need to learn to enhance self-control by focusing attention on their goals,[47] activate problem-solving processes to deal with competing goals,[48] and develop appropriate self-talk for stages before, during, and after the challenging situation (stress inoculation).[27]

Communicating assertively

Communication skills are needed in a variety of situations to maximize support, confront obstacles, and minimize negative social influences. Situations requiring assertiveness skills include saying no to unhealthy social behaviors, making specific dietary requests at a restaurant, and asking for help from family members.

Element 4: Environmental Resources

Resource use includes securing medication, supplies, and educational resources.[49] The best efforts of self-management will be defeated if there is no access to the necessary supplies from the environment, or if the environment contains pernicious elements. For example, if people living with HIV lack access to antiretroviral drugs, their illness becomes acute and terminal rather than a chronic disease that can be effectively self-managed. Environmental barriers to obtaining resources (eg, transportation issues) and maintaining healthy behaviors (eg, safe settings for exercise) require action plans to overcome them. Part of self-management is to be aware of, and take concerted action to avoid, environmental settings that derail goal attainment, and to use problem-solving skills to develop and achieve action plans.

Recommendations for environmental structuring[50] and principles of environmental control[8] are included in many SMIs. In behavior modification, environment is relevant as a source of situational cues and a potent reinforcer for both positive and negative behaviors. The self-managing patient is advised to create a home environment with stimuli for healthy behaviors (eg, fruits and vegetables in the refrigerator; treadmill in front of the television), take steps to remove stimuli for problematic behavior (eg, junk food, alcohol), and seek healthy environments while avoiding unhealthy environments (eg, gyms vs fast food restaurants).

Element 5: Social Support

The current approach to SMI may overemphasize individual variables such as self-efficacy and neglect the importance of social factors.[51] Supportive relationships have been identified as an important component in interventions to promote healthy behaviors,[52] and good self-managers have extensive support networks.[53] Health-promoting decisions can be both supported or impeded by family and friends. Negative influences can come from well-intentioned people, as when they reinforce a sick role instead of supporting the autonomy and empowerment of the patient. Cultural norms and values need to be addressed to ensure optimum social support.[27,54] Health providers are an essential source of encouragement, positive reinforcement, and emotional support.

DEVELOPMENT OF SELF-MANAGEMENT COMPETENCE

Competence in self-management occurs over time, in phases. Interventions should be targeted to the appropriate stage[45] and meet patients at their current level of information and skills.[39] **Fig. 1** presents a 3-phase model that shows the patient's journey to a healthy lifestyle. This figure simplifies the process of developing competence, which

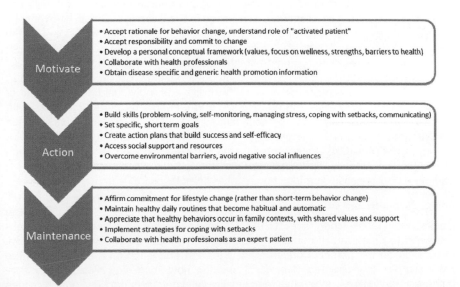

Fig. 1. Patient process of developing self-management.

is best viewed as iterative and cyclical, as the patient makes progress on subgoals at different rates, and will inevitably experience new challenges over time, requiring a return to the motivation phase. Despite that limitation, this model illustrates the different outcomes—knowledge, attitudes, and skills—at different stages in the trajectory of choosing healthy behaviors, and may help determine the best delivery vehicle for self-management interventions.

DELIVERY VEHICLES FOR SELF-MANAGEMENT INTERVENTIONS

The diffusion of interventions that promote successful self-management is essential for improving health-related quality of life, reducing health care costs over time, and preventing the progression of chronic conditions. This section reviews delivery vehicles with varying levels of expense and professional involvement for promoting self-management. As new delivery vehicles are developed, interventions can be tailored to the cultural and social needs of individuals, wider dissemination will be possible, and gaps in one form of delivery will be filled by the services of another.

Primary Care Settings

The Chronic Care Model (CCM) requires a major rethinking of primary care practice, with nonphysician personnel trained to support patient self-management, and new, collaborative roles for health care professionals.[9] While behavioral interventions in the medical office are effective, and interventions introduced by a physician garner greater participation,[55] patients participate in clinical decisions only 9% of the time, pointing to the need for physicians to learn skills for group facilitation, problem-solving, goal-setting, and cognitive–behavioral techniques.[17]

Group Interventions

There are many successful evidence-based group interventions for chronic illness that promote behavioral self-management, yet these interventions are not broadly diffused in the United States; they are typically delivered only for a few diseases (eg, diabetes), and are usually implemented only when diseases become chronic and debilitating rather than as strategies of primary and secondary prevention. Group interventions are often led by peers (expert patients who have received special training) or health professionals such as nurses and dieticians.[54]

There are drawbacks to relying on standardized self-management group interventions as the sole means of developing competent patients. Critics of the UK Expert Patients Program complain that it lacks flexibility and individualization because of requirements to adhere to rigid protocols,[53] and it should be better integrated with primary care and attend more to social factors.[51] Lack of participation and attrition are barriers to success,[40,54] especially when support for the maintenance of behavior change is not provided. Group programs rarely provide support for the maintenance phase (the final stage in the stages of change model), with the exception of a program offering a booster session a few months after completion.[54,56]

Books, Manuals, and Other Media

Books, audio tapes, video tapes, CD-ROMs, and self-directed manuals can be effective ways to promote self-management,[57] with or without an in-person intervention, depending on the personal preferences, age, and education level of the audience. For example, Self-directed Behavior[58] teaches how to design step-by-step self-change interventions, integrates empirically validated approaches, and provides guidelines for how to revise plans when strategies are unsuccessful.

Disease Management Companies

Commercial disease management companies offer financial savings and improved health, generally through increased use of care managers rather than the systematic teaching of skills of self-management.[59] American Healthways, the largest disease management company, provides a program with health coaching, patient education, and phone calls to patients, including a virtual health coach project that integrates information therapy and behavior change interventions based on the stages of change model.[60]

Individual or Family Coaching Sessions

Another delivery vehicle is individual coaching with a health educator or counselor (alone or in combination with other methods), or one-on-one sessions and individual follow-ups as a supplement to the core program. Individual coaching or counseling provides added motivation, time to address an individual's specific barriers or challenges, opportunities to include family members as social support, and enhancement of an individual's capacity for self-control.

Technological Innovations

Web sites, E-mail, and touch-screen computers offer tools for self-management.[55,61,62] One example is Diabetes Prevention Source (DPS) Health's Behavior Change Suite, a Web-based platform that incorporates key behavior change strategies in an online, interactive experience that includes goal setting, self-monitoring, visual feedback on progress over time, automated reminders, physical activity monitoring with integrated accelerometers, virtual real-time or message-based coaching, interactive lessons, streaming audio and video, and social support and networking features. Interactive voice response (IVR), mobile phones, and text messages also facilitate self-monitoring through data collection, monitoring and reporting of blood glucose level (for diabetics), positive reinforcement messages, and reminders for medication and behavior adherence.[63,64] Mobile personal sensing (MPS) offers the opportunity for broadly accessible, privacy-preserving ecological momentary assessment (EMA), the self-report of symptoms, behaviors, feelings, and cognitions the moment that they occur.[65] MPS is moving toward technology for biosensors to monitor physiologic health data, collect information for activity classification, and provide notifications for problematic contexts and locations.[66] EMA has been used for self-monitoring to change behaviors related to drug and alcohol use, coping with chronic pain, and stress and cardiovascular reactivity.[67]

SUMMARY

There has been little consensus on the components of SMIs that are most effective, but the authors' 5-element, 3-phase framework can be used to evaluate currently implemented SMIs, identify gaps in interventions, and identify each patient's strengths and deficits for personalized interventions. Self-management is applicable to primary prevention for healthy people as well as the health and lifestyle improvement of the chronically ill.

Self-management approaches are more economical than traditional disease management because professional roles can be filled by health educators and counselors rather than physicians. Moreover, they can take place in community settings, on the Internet, or by phone to lessen the demand on overburdened medical settings.[17] It is predicted that patients who adhere to healthy lifestyles and habitually use self-management tools will be protected from the severe symptoms that require hospital use, a major contributor to high health care costs. Currently, no long-term follow-up research has been completed to demonstrate that SMI significantly reduces health care costs over an extended period of time.

Shifting responsibility of some aspects of health management to patients requires a change in how provider and patient roles are viewed by both. However, self-management does not mean the exclusion of health professionals. Rather, it represents a new model of active collaboration between expert patients and patient-centered practitioners. Self-management interventions will result in decreased burden on the overall health care system and will support more optimized use of limited resources. Additionally, it will increase a patient's investment in, and responsibility for, his or her own care. Health care professionals will have roles in both education of self-management methods and ongoing support for maintenance of results. Personnel with less education, such as community health workers (CHWs), will be necessary for providing adjunctive support, basic follow-up and feedback, positive reinforcement, and accountability. Primary care providers can support patient self-management by encouraging patients to become more informed, active, and responsible in the provider–patient relationship, and by trusting patients to be experts on their symptoms and health condition, particularly the longer the patient has coped with the condition.

Health policy changes will be necessary to make self-management a priority and provide funds for training, employment, technology development, and dissemination. Most importantly, there should be a termination of the sharp division between prevention and disease management that is evident in the structure and missions of different government agencies. As a solution to the staggering costs of chronic disease, DeVol and colleagues[6] propose incentives for prevention and early intervention through private–public partnerships, and a national commitment to promote health and wellness.

A family wellness model offers the best potential for sustained improvement in global health, by going beyond a disease management model to instill healthy behaviors at the level of the family as primary prevention.[68] Ultimately, the solution to the high human and financial cost of chronic illnesses will be health-promoting families, with each member, regardless of health status, committed to eating well, keeping active, avoiding alcohol and tobacco, and embracing stress-reducing behaviors through the self-management of healthy living.

REFERENCES

1. California Health Care Foundation. California health care almanac: health care costs 101. 2011. Available at: http://www.chcf.org/~/media/MEDIA%20LIBRARY%20Files/PDF/H/PDF%20HealthCareCosts11.pdf. Accessed March 5, 2011.
2. Central Intelligence Agency. The world factbook. Updated February 15, 2012. Available at: https://www.cia.gov/library/publications/the-world-factbook/rankorder/2102rank.html. Accessed March 5, 2012.
3. Paez KA, Zhao L, Hwang W. Rising out-of-pocket spending for chronic conditions: a ten-year trend. Health Aff 2009;28(1):15–25.
4. Bodenheimer T, Chen E, Bennett HD. Confronting the growing burden of chronic disease: can the U.S. health care workforce do the job? Health Aff 2009;28(1):64–74.
5. Foote SM. Next steps: how can Medicare accelerate the pace of improving chronic care? Health Aff 2009;28:99–102.
6. DeVol R, Bedroussian A, Charuworn A, et al. An unhealthy America: the economic burden of chronic disease—charting a new course to save lives and increase productivity and economic growth. Santa Monica (CA): Milken Institute; 2007.

7. World Health Organization. 2008–2013 Action plan for the global strategy for the prevention and control of noncommunicable diseases. 2009. Available at: http://www.who.int/chp/action/en/. Accessed July 14, 2009.
8. Bodenheimer T, Lorig K, Holman H, et al. Patient self-management of chronic disease in primary care. JAMA 2002;288(19):2469–75.
9. Bodenheimer T, Wagner EH, Grumbach K. Improving primary care for patients with chronic illness. JAMA 2002;288(14):1775–9.
10. Epping-Jordan J, Bengoa R, Kawar R, et al. The challenge of chronic conditions: WHO responds. BMJ 2001;323:947–8.
11. Creer TL, Holroyd KA, Glasgow RE, et al. Health psychology (chapter 15). In: Lambert MJ, editor. Bergin and Garfield's handbook of psychotherapy and behavior change. 5th edition. New York: John Wiley & Sons; 2004. p. 697–742.
12. Purdie N, McCrindle A. Self-regulation, self-efficacy and health behavior change in older adults. Educ Gerontol 2002;28(5):379–400.
13. Glasgow RE, Toobert DJ, Barrera M, et al. Assessment of problem-solving: a key to successful diabetes self-management. J Behav Med 2004;27(5):477–90.
14. Chodosh J, Morton SC, Mojica W, et al. Meta-analysis: chronic disease self-management programs for older adults. Ann Intern Med 2005;143:427–38.
15. Rasmussen HN, Wrosch C, Scheier MF, et al. Self-regulation processes and health: the importance of optimism and goal adjustment. J Pers 2006;74(6): 1721–47.
16. Schwarzer R. Social–cognitive factors in changing health-related behaviors. Curr Dir Psychol Sci 2001;10(2):47–51.
17. Newman S, Steed L, Mulligan K. Self-management interventions for chronic illness. Lancet 2004;364:1523–37.
18. Barlow JH, Wright CC, Sheasby JE, et al. Self-management approaches for people with chronic conditions: a review. Patient Educ Couns 2002;48: 177–87.
19. Nolte S, Elsworth GR, Sinclair AJ, et al. The extent and breadth of benefits from participating in chronic disease self-management courses: a national patient-reported outcomes survey. Patient Educ Couns 2007;65(3):351–60.
20. Warsi A, Wang PS, LaValley MP, et al. Self-management education programs in chronic disease: a systematic review and methodological critique of the literature. Arch Intern Med 2004;164:1641–9.
21. Fisher EB, Brownson CA, O'Toole ML, et al. Ecological approaches to self-management: the case of diabetes. Am J Public Health 2005;95(9):1523–35.
22. Jerant AF, von Friederichs-Fitzwater MM, Moore M. Patients' perceived barriers to active self-management of chronic conditions. Patient Educ Couns 2005;57: 300–7.
23. Lorig K, Holman H. Self-management education: history, definition, outcomes and mechanisms. Ann Behav Med 2003;26(1):1–7.
24. Swendeman D, Ingram BL, Rotheram-Borus MJ. Common elements in self-management of HIV and other chronic illnesses: an integrative framework. AIDS Care 2009;21(10):1321–34.
25. Anderson RM. Patient empowerment and the traditional medical model: a case of irreconcilable differences? Diabetes Care 1995;18:412–5.
26. Aujoulat I, d'Hoore W, Deccache A. Patient empowerment in theory and practice: polysemy or cacophony? Patient Educ Couns 2007;66(1):13–20.
27. Karoly P, Boekaerts M, Maes S. Toward consensus in the psychology of self-regulation: how far have we come? How far do we have yet to travel? Int Rev Appl Psychol 2005;54(2):300–11.

28. Prochaska JO, DiClemente CC. Stages and processes of self-change of smoking: toward an integrative model of change. J Consult Clin Psychol 1983; 51:390–5.
29. Cassidy CA. Using the transtheoretical model to facilitate behavior change in patients with chronic illness. J Am Acad Nurse Pract 1999;11:281–7.
30. Kerns RD, Rosenberg R. Predicting responses to self-management treatments for chronic pain: application of the pain stages of change model. Pain 2000;84: 49–55.
31. Miller WR, Rollnick S. Motivational interviewing: preparing people to change addictive behavior. New York: Guilford Press; 1991.
32. Britt E, Hudson SM, Blampied NM. Motivational interviewing in health settings: a review. Patient Educ Couns 2004;53:147–55.
33. Knight KM, McGowan L, Dickens C, et al. A systematic review of motivational interviewing in physical health care settings. Br J Health Psychol 2006;11(2): 319–32.
34. Bellg AJ. Maintenance of health behavior change in preventive cardiology: internalization and self-regulation of new behaviors. Behav Modif 2003;27: 103–31.
35. Wilde MH, Garvin S. A concept analysis of self-monitoring. J Adv Nurs 2007; 57(3):339–50.
36. Maes S, Gebhardt W. Self-regulation and health behavior: the health behavior goal model. In: Boekaerts M, Pintrich PR, Zeidner M, editors. Handbook of self-regulation. Burlington (MA): Elsevier Academic Press; 2000. p. 343–68.
37. Uchino BM, Cacioppo JT, Kiecolt-Glaser JK. The relationship between social support and physiological process: a review with emphasis on underlying mechanisms and implications for health. Psychol Bull 1996;119:488–531.
38. Gifford AL, Sengupta S. Self-management health education for chronic HIV infection. AIDS Care 1999;11(1):115–30.
39. Skinner TC, Carey ME, Cradock S, et al. Diabetes education and self-management for ongoing and newly diagnosed (DESMOND): process modeling of pilot study. Patient Educ Couns 2006;64:369–77.
40. Clark M, Hampson SE, Avery L, et al. Effects of a brief tailored intervention on the process and predictors of lifestyle behaviour change in patients with type 2 diabetes. Psychol Health Med 2004;9(4):440–9.
41. Wright CC, Barlow JH, Turner AP, et al. Self-management training for people with chronic disease: an exploratory study. Br J Health Psychol 2003;8(4): 465–76.
42. Mossavar-Rahmani Y, Henry H, Rodabough R, et al. Additional self-monitoring tools in the dietary modification component of the women's health initiative. J Am Diet Assoc 2004;104(1):76–85.
43. Charmaz K. Good days, bad days: the self in chronic illness and time. New Brunswick (NJ): Rutgers University Press; 1991.
44. Bayliss EA, Ellis JL, Steiner JF. Barriers to self-management and quality-of-life outcomes in seniors with mutimorbidities. Ann Fam Med 2007;5:395–402.
45. Hibbard JH, Mahoney ER, Stock R, et al. Self-management and health care utilization: do increases in patient activation result in improved self-management behaviors? Health Serv Res 2007;42(4):1443–63.
46. Witkiewitz K, Marlatt GA. Relapse prevention for alcohol and drug problems: that was zen, this is tao. Am Psychol 2004;59:224–35.
47. Metcalfe J, Mischel W. A hot/cool-system analysis of delay of gratification: dynamics of willpower. Psychol Rev 1999;106:3–19.

48. Leventhal H, Mora PA. Is there a science of the processes underlying health and illness behaviors? A comment on Maes and Karoly. Int Rev Appl Psychol 2005; 54(2):255–66.
49. Nagelkerk J, Reick K, Meengs L. Perceived barriers and effective strategies to diabetes self-management. J Adv Nurs 2006;54(2):151–8.
50. Kitsantas A. The role of self-regulation strategies and self-efficacy perceptions in successful weight loss maintenance. Psychol Health 2000;15(6):811–20.
51. Taylor D, Bury M. Chronic illness, expert patients and care transition. Sociol Health Illn 2007;29:27–45.
52. Bull S, Eakin E, Reevers M, et al. Multi-level support for physical activity and healthy eating. J Adv Nurs 2006;54(5):585–93.
53. MacDonald W, Rogers A, Blakeman T, et al. Practice nurses and the facilitation of self-management in primary care. J Adv Nurs 2008;62(2):191–9.
54. Steed L, Lankester J, Barnard M, et al. Evaluation of the UCL Diabetes Self-Management Programme (UCL-DSMP): a randomized controlled trial. J Health Psychol 2005;10:261–75.
55. Glasgow RE, LaChance PA, Toobert DJ, et al. Long-term effects and costs of brief behavioural dietary interventions for patients with diabetes delivered from the medical office. Patient Educ Couns 1997;32:175–84.
56. Clifford PA, Tan SY, Gorsuch RL. Efficacy of a self-directed behavioral health change program: weight, body composition, cardiovascular fitness, blood pressure, health risk, and psychosocial mediating variables. J Behav Med 1991;14: 303–23.
57. Janevic MR, Janz NK, Dodge JA, et al. The role of choice in health education intervention trials: a review and case study. Soc Sci Med 2003;56:1581–94.
58. Watson DL, Tharp RG. Self-directed behavior. 9th edition. Belmont (CA): Wadsworth Publishing Company; 2007.
59. Crosson FJ, Madvig P. Does population management of chronic disease lead to lower costs of care? Health Aff 2004;23(6):76–8.
60. American Healthways. Center for Information Therapy to jointly develop Ix best practices. The Free Library; 2005. Available at: http://www.thefreelibrary.com/ American Healthways. Accessed August 3, 2009.
61. Lorig K. What are the barriers to healthcare systems using a biopsychosocial approach and how might they be overcome?. In: White P, editor. Biopsychosocial medicine: an integrated approach to understanding illness. New York: Oxford University Press; 2005. p. 201–15.
62. Tate DF, Wing RR, Winett RA. Using Internet technology to deliver a behavioral weight loss program. JAMA 2001;285:1172–7.
63. Bardone AM, Krahn DD, Goodman BM, et al. Using interactive voice response technology and timeline follow-back methodology in studying binge eating and drinking behavior: different answers to different forms of the same question? Addict Behav 2000;25:1–11.
64. Fjeldsoe BS, Marshall AL, Miller YD. Behavior change interventions delivered by mobile telephone short-message service. Am J Prev Med 2009;36(2):165–73.
65. Moscowitz DS, Young SN. Ecological momentary assessment: what it is and why it is a method of the future in clinical psychopharmacology. J Psychiatry Neurosci 2006;31(1):13–20.
66. Ramanathan N, Burke J, Cenizal CJ, et al. Improving personal and environmental health decision making with mobile personal sensing (May 12, 2009). Center for Embedded Network Sensing; 2009. Posters. Paper 430. Available at: http:// repositories.cdlib.org/cens/Posters/430. Accessed June 23, 2009.

67. Freedman MJ, Lester KM, McNamara C, et al. Cell phones for ecological momentary assessment with cocaine-addicted homeless patients in treatment. J Subst Abuse Treat 2006;30(2):105–11.
68. Rotheram-Borus MJ, Swendeman D, Flannery D. Family wellness, not HIV prevention. AIDS Behav 2009;13:409–13.

Optimizing Pain Management Through Collaborations with Behavioral and Addiction Medicine in Primary Care

Matthew Brensilver, PhD, Shabana Tariq, MD,
Steven Shoptaw, PhD*

KEYWORDS

- Chronic noncancer pain • Opioids • Interdisciplinary
- Patient-centered medical home • Addiction

KEY POINTS

- Chronic noncancer pain (CNCP) affects a high proportion of primary care patients, and carries a large human and economic burden. In response to the widespread perception that pain has been underdiagnosed and undertreated, regulatory bodies have encouraged more comprehensive services to address pain syndromes.
- Significant hurdles exist in treating CNCP in primary care settings, including a relative lack of training, lower physician satisfaction in treating pain patients, lack of objective measures, and the risks associated with opioid treatment including addiction. In addition, interventional therapies and pharmacotherapy often do not provide complete symptomatic relief.
- The utility of collaborations with behavioral and addiction medicine specialists optimizes care and advances models of patient treatment within a primary care patient-centered medical home.

Pain is an important signal that something is wrong with our bodies, which confers unambiguous adaptive functions. Pain signals to the body mean that tissue damage has occurred that needs repair and/or alerts the individual to environmental threats to survival. Indeed, those with a rare, genetically mediated syndrome whereby pain is not experienced face significant functional impairments that can be life threatening.[1] In chronic illnesses, however, pain may linger despite limited or even no adaptive

---

Conflicts of interest: All authors report no conflicts of interest.
Funding: The authors acknowledge the support of NIDA grants P50 DA-18185 and T32 DA026400.
Department of Family Medicine, David Geffen School of Medicine at UCLA, CA 90095, USA
* Corresponding author. Steven Shoptaw 10880 Wilshire Boulevard, Suite 1800, Los Angeles, CA.
E-mail address: sshoptaw@mednet.ucla.edu

signal for the individual. This situation is encountered frequently in primary care as the prevalence of chronic diseases increases in the American population, and acute pain in the context of chronic disease impairs functioning and contributes to human suffering. Moreover, as patients repeatedly seek medical care to reduce their pain, providers become frustrated by limited progress when prescribing powerful analgesics to their patients with chronic noncancer pain (CNCP). This article discusses existing approaches in primary care that are designed to help patients to better manage CNCP, with particular emphasis on implementation of these efforts in the context of behavioral and addiction medicine. CNCP and addiction are chronic diseases that provide opportunities to integrate these conditions within the patient-centered medical home framework. Furthermore, a team-based program developed to address these conditions within an academic primary care clinic has used the building blocks of high-performing primary care clinics identified by Willard and Bodenheimer,[2] which include data-driven improvements, managing panel size, team-based care, population management, continuity of care, and prompt access to care.

In 2001, The Joint Commission (TJC) established pain-management standards for accredited ambulatory care facilities, behavioral health care organizations, hospitals, home care, and long-term care facilities. These standards require that patients be assessed and treated for pain, and encourage patients to report pain to their providers. The action of TJC was a response to the widespread perception that pain had been underdiagnosed and undertreated. Similar actions were taken within the Veterans Administration health care system, which is creating a comprehensive, system-wide approach to pain management that ensures the active assessment and treatment of chronic pain.[3]

The establishment of pain as the "fifth vital sign" is justified by a cursory examination of the prevalence of chronic pain. Although there is no universally accepted definition of chronic pain, it is commonly defined as pain persisting beyond the time for normal tissue healing, typically specified between 3 and 6 months. This article limits its attention to CNCP, which presents additional challenges when compared with pain related to malignancies. In a nationally representative sample of 27,035 in the United States, the crude point prevalence of pain lasting at least 6 months is 34.5%.[4] Adjusted for the population characteristics of the nation, prevalence is estimated at 30.7%. Chronic pain increases across age groups, and is more prevalent among women (34.3%) than men (26.7%). Chronic low back pain is the most commonly reported pain syndrome. Prevalence rates for pediatric populations vary widely, but even low estimates suggest a substantial burden on this population.[5] The Institute of Medicine (IOM) recently issued a report titled *Relieving Pain in America: A Blueprint for Transforming Prevention, Care, Education and Research*. The report estimates that 100 million Americans suffer from chronic pain,[6] a figure that closely coheres with other epidemiologic estimates.[4,7]

Chronic pain exerts an enormous public health burden. A nationally representative survey of 28,902 working adults assessed the economic impacts created by pain conditions.[8] Over one-half (53%) of these individuals admitted to having pain in the 2-week period before the survey. Thirteen percent lost productive time as a result of the pain. Absence days were uncommon, and most productivity loss was due to reduced performance on the job. Among those with low back pain, direct costs for medical care are estimated to be US$26 billion.[9] On average, individuals with back pain incurred health care expenditures about 60% higher than individuals without back pain ($3498 vs $2178) and in the report from the IOM, the total estimated annual economic cost of chronic pain in the United States is between $560 and $635 billion. This estimate reflects the combined cost of health care ($261–$300 billion) and the cost of lost productivity ($297–$336 billion) associated with chronic pain. The investigators suggest that these estimates are likely conservative, as it excludes the cost of pain associated with institutionalized individuals, children, and military personnel. Pain is associated with clinically important comorbidities,[10] including a 4-fold increase in odds of having an anxiety or depressive disorder.[11]

The American College of Physicians and the American Pain Society issued a joint clinical guideline for the diagnosis and treatment of low back pain.[12] It is reported that low back pain is the fifth most common reason for all physician visits in the United States. One survey by the World Health Organization screened 25,619 primary care patients in 14 countries and found that 22% (range: 6%–33%) reported pain persisting longer than 6 months.[11] Primary care physicians are responsible for a substantial proportion of the care for chronic pain.[13] Yet in a survey of primary care resident physicians, more than one-half rated their medical school preparation for treatment of chronic, noncancer pain as poor or fair, with similar dissatisfactions expressed with residency training.[14] Treating CNCP can be wearisome; physicians report a lack of confidence in their ability to treat pain effectively and have aversive responses to the treatment challenges.[15–17] Primary care physicians face barriers to providing care for chronic pain including lack of objective measures of pain, lack of expertise in treating chronic pain, coexisting disorders including addiction, aberrant patient behaviors, and legal complications associated with prescribing opioids.[18] The role of primary care physicians is often to assist patients with self-management strategies, but many lack the training to confidently perform such a role, and reimbursement structures provide little incentive for providing this type of care.[6]

As expected, patients with CNCP represent a common population in primary care settings, are expensive as measured by human and economic burden, and are often difficult to treat without the support of a team with the understanding of this special-needs population. The development of a multidisciplinary team of specialists coupled with a front and back office staff prepared to address the unique needs of this population has been developed in the authors' academic primary care health center. A collaborative interdisciplinary model has been implemented and evaluated to address barriers for payment to pain, addiction, and behavioral medicine physicians for services that become the responsibility of the primary care provider, particularly for those health plans aimed at providing care to underinsured populations. Furthermore, panel size, roles and responsibilities of team members, and length of treatment ensure both continuity of care and prompt access to care. For most patients with CNCP, a credentialed pain medicine physician serves as a consultant as well as primary care provider until alternative diagnoses are made or the patient is stabilized and subsequently transferred to the family physician for ongoing care. The pain medicine physician collaborates with the family physician and the specialists from the Behavioral Medicine Clinic (BMED) and Addiction Medicine Clinic (AMED). Established relationships with physical therapy clinics provide easy referral paths for patients who might benefit. This integrated care provides a single home for many pain patients. In what follows, the rationale and implementation of an interdisciplinary model of pain treatment is described.

INTERDISCIPLINARY MODEL OF PAIN TREATMENT
Collaborations with the Behavioral Medicine Clinic

Despite advances in interventional therapies, surgery, and pharmacotherapy for chronic pain, symptomatic relief is often incomplete.[19] Even when these therapies provide relief from the experience of pain, functional improvements are often not witnessed. The purely biomedical model has been largely replaced by a bio-psychosocial model whereby the experience and burden of pain reflect the dynamic interplay of physiologic, psychological, and social factors.[10] The transition from acute injury to chronic pain related disability is predicted by a range of psychosocial variables including maladaptive beliefs, lack of social support, depressive mood, and somatization.[20,21] Psychosocial and behavioral factors contribute significantly to the experience, maintenance, and exacerbation of pain.[19] The American Pain Society guidelines for treatment of chronic low back pain recommend that patients with non-radicular pain receive interdisciplinary treatment if first-line treatments fail to resolve the symptoms.[12] Although modest in their effects, several reviews highlight the effectiveness of behavioral treatments.[10,22,23] A recent meta-analysis examined the efficacy of psychological interventions for chronic low back pain and found reductions in self-reported pain, depression, and disability, and increases in quality of life.[24]

Short-term, cognitive-behaviorally focused approaches to management of CNCP can help patients address functional and psychological problems that arise over their chronic illnesses.[25,26] Within the context of a behavioral medicine clinic, elements of these approaches in behavioral medicine sessions that correspond with functional improvement include the following. (1) An increasing ability to tolerate distress caused by mild to moderate levels of pain to fulfill roles for family and job. This approach can include cognitive (eg, identifying and challenging negative cognitions) and behavioral (eg, diaphragmatic breathing, mindfulness) methods. (2) Deemphasizing the role for analgesic medications as the central element for managing pain. (3) Helping patients to become more physically active in all spheres of their life, while respecting their limits. (4) Educating family members and enlisting their involvement in supporting efforts to increase functional abilities. (5) Working with the health system to discourage medication-seeking behaviors, especially frequent use of emergency departments to access opioid analgesics.

As the offices for pain and behavioral medicine are colocated, coordination between the pain specialist and psychologist is straightforward. Typically the pain physician will provide a referral for an assessment and possibly brief treatment to one of the clinicians in BMED. The pain medicine physician meets directly with a clinician from BMED to discuss the patient and provide treatment recommendations. When indicated, BMED staff and the pain specialist meet jointly with the patient. As the patient's primary care physician is on staff at the health center, coordinating care is uncomplicated. Referrals flow in both directions. Cases within behavioral medicine frequently are complex, involving disorders or diseases that will not improve and that involve pain problems that are challenging to manage using pharmacotherapy only. In collaboration with the primary care physician, BMED can facilitate closer pain management by the primary care physician or provide a referral to the pain specialist.

Intersection of Pain Treatment and Addiction Medicine

Pain medicine clinics almost invariably intersect with addiction treatment. This section describes opioid-prescribing trends and some of the unintended negative consequences of increased accessibility of prescription opioids. These data highlight the importance of close collaboration between pain clinics and addiction medicine specialists.

Over the past 2 decades, the recognition of the scope and urgency of pain has led to dramatic increases in opioid-prescribing rates.[27] In 1997, the morphine-equivalent dose prescribed, per person, was 100 mg. By 2007, this figure had risen to 700 mg.[28] As of 2005, approximately 10 million Americans were receiving chronic opioid therapy (COT).[29] More aggressive treatment of pain has alleviated suffering but carries unintended negative consequences. Those at elevated risk for opioid misuse, such as individuals with comorbid psychiatric disorders, are more likely to be prescribed opioid medications.[30] Younger individuals and those with prior substance-abuse problems are also at higher risk for misuse, and receive opioids at elevated rates.[31]

The National Survey on Drug Use and Health, a representative sample of 92,000, found 4.5% of adults reported nonmedical use of prescription opioids in past year.[32] In the most recent annual data available, 2.2 million people initiated illicit use of opioids, with only marijuana exceeding opioids as the substance associated with illicit drug initiation.[33] Between 2004 and 2009 the number of emergency room visits for misuse of prescription drugs doubled, with opioid-related problems figuring prominently in this increase.[34] Oxycodone-related emergency department visits increased 242% during this period with substantial increases also noted for hydrocodone, morphine, and fentanyl. These patterns have been paralleled by disturbing trends in opioid-related poisonings. Poisoning is the second leading cause of accidental death in the United States, and more than one-third of all poisonings involve opioid medications.[35] Fatal overdoses increased overall, but involvement of opioids increased dramatically, climbing from 21% in 1999 to 37% in 2006, an increase of 76%.

Although opioid medications are often obtained through illegal means, legitimate physicians' prescriptions figure prominently in opioid misuse and its associated morbidity and mortality. In nationally representative data from 2006 through 2008, Becker and colleagues[36] found that of those misusing opioids, 31% had a physician source and approximately 20% were receiving opioids exclusively from their physician. The situation led the President's Office of National Drug Control Policy to release a recent report entitled *Epidemic: Responding to America's Prescription Drug Abuse Crisis*.

Despite the risks associated with opioid treatment, the prescribing practices of primary care providers are not optimal. Among fully trained primary care physicians, opioid risk-reduction strategies are not commonly implemented. Starrels and colleagues[37] assessed the use of risk-reduction strategies among primary care physicians caring for patients on continuous opioid therapy. Only 8% of patients ever submitted a urine drug screen, 50% failed to have regular monitoring visits, and 77% received repeated early refills. Of individuals with multiple risk factors for opioid misuse, risk strategies were not implemented at higher rates, and in some cases were actually implemented less frequently for those at greatest risk.

While the majority of patients in the authors' pain clinic can safely use opioids and adhere to physician directions, a significant minority shows signs of problematic use. Rates of aberrant drug-taking behavior vary widely,[38] but one systematic review estimated a rate of 11.5%.[39] Before initiating opioid treatment, the pain clinic stratifies the risk level according to a range of factors predictive of opioid misuse including a personal or family history of substance abuse, younger age, and comorbid psychiatric disorder.[40,41] For higher-risk patients more stringent and more frequent monitoring is provided, in accord with recent guidelines for COT for CNCP.[41] These monitoring strategies include risk-assessment questionnaires such as the Current Opioid Misuse Measure[40] opioid contracts, more frequent visits, withholding any requests for early refills, prescription drug monitoring program reports, and urine drug screening.

Despite these efforts, a small minority of patients develop use indicative not merely of physiologic dependence that develops with COT[42] but a loss of control over drug taking. Here, collaboration with AMED becomes essential. Often the pain physician will consult with the addiction medicine physician and, when appropriate, meet jointly with the patient. If the problematic use of opioids does not resolve quickly, the team might consider induction onto buprenorphine-naloxone (Suboxone). Buprenorphine is a partial agonist that binds tightly to μ-opioid receptors, but features low intrinsic activity. This combination of properties blocks the euphoric effects of full agonists while attenuating craving and withdrawal symptoms. Its effectiveness in opioid addiction is well established.[43,44] Although indicated for maintenance treatment of opioid dependence, for mild to moderate pain high doses of buprenorphine will have some analgesic effects, although pain relief may be incomplete. Dosing may need to be more frequent than is typical with buprenorphine, as its analgesic effects are shorter acting than the suppression of opioid craving and withdrawal symptoms.

A case series of 95 CNCP patients attests to the therapeutic effects of buprenorphine in this population.[45] There are some guidelines that have been offered for the treatment of acute pain in the context of methadone or buprenorphine patients.[46] In this case, the investigators warn against common misconceptions that lead to the undertreatment of pain for patients on opioid substitution therapy. Flexibility in the treatment approach for acute pain is feasible. However, negotiating the challenge of a bona fide chronic pain condition in the context opioid addiction is complex, and minimal empiric data exist to guide decision making. Blondell and colleagues[47] assessed buprenorphine for individuals with CNCP and comorbid opioid addiction. The trial was terminated prematurely, as none of the 6 participants assigned to a 4-month buprenorphine taper condition completed the trial. Of those continuing with buprenorphine treatment and a 6-month follow-up, the majority reported increased functioning and persistent analgesic effects of the medication. An adaptive trial design recently assessed buprenorphine-naloxone in opioid-dependent patients.[48] Although patients with severe chronic pain were excluded from the trial, those with mild to moderate pain comprised 42% of the sample. A brief stabilization with buprenorphine followed by behavioral support failed the vast majority of participants in terms of opioid abstinence. Those failing treatment were enrolled in the second phase of the trial, and all received extended buprenorphine-naloxone treatment. Success at the end of treatment was much greater than outcomes from the first phase, with 49.2% abstinent from opioids. Of relevance, chronic pain did not moderate treatment outcomes, suggesting that the use of buprenorphine-naloxone is similar in patients with and without mild to moderate chronic pain.

SUMMARY

CNCP figures prominently in the health of primary care patients, and carries an enormous human and economic burden. The recognition that pain has been underdiagnosed and undertreated has encouraged more comprehensive services to meet the needs of these patients. Despite its prevalence, organizational and therapeutic challenges exist in treating CNCP in primary care settings. Interventional therapies and pharmacotherapy often do not provide complete symptomatic relief. At the University of California Los Angeles Family Health Center, the authors have created an interdisciplinary pain clinic that includes a pain physician working in collaboration with behavioral and addiction medicine specialists. This approach helps to successfully address the multidimensional nature of chronic pain conditions, and provides confidence that the complexities arising from chronic opioid treatment can be managed effectively.

REFERENCES

1. Cox JJ, Reimann F, Nicholas AK, et al. An SCN9A channelopathy causes congenital inability to experience pain. Nature 2006;444:894–8.
2. Willard R, Bodenheimer T. The building blocks of high-performing primary care: lessons from the field. California Healthcare Foundation; 2012.

3. Department of Veterans Affairs. VHA Directive 2009-053: pain management. October 28, 2009. Available at: http://www.va.gov/PAINMANAGEMENT/docs/VHA09PainDirective.pdf. Accessed July 3, 2012.

4. Johannes CB, Le TK, Zhou X, et al. The prevalence of chronic pain in United States adults: results of an internet-based survey. J Pain 2010;11:1230–9.

5. Vetter TR. The epidemiology of pediatric chronic pain. Handbook of pediatric chronic pain 2011;1–14.

6. Institute of Medicine. Relieving pain in America: blueprint for transforming prevention, care, education, and research. Washington, DC: National Academies Press; 2011.

7. Munce SE, Stewart DE. Gender differences in depression and chronic pain conditions in a national epidemiologic survey. Psychosomatics 2007;48:394–9.

8. Stewart WF, Ricci JA, Chee E, et al. Lost productive time and cost due to common pain conditions in the US workforce. JAMA 2003;290:2443–54.

9. Luo X, Pietrobon R, Sun SX, et al. Estimates and patterns of direct health care expenditures among individuals with back pain in the United States. Spine 2004;29:79–86.

10. Gatchel RJ, Peng YB, Peters ML, et al. The biopsychosocial approach to chronic pain: scientific advances and future directions. Psychol Bull 2007;133:581–624.

11. Gureje O, Von Korff M, Simon GE, et al. Persistent pain and well-being. JAMA 1998;280:147–51.

12. Chou R, Qaseem A, Snow V, et al. Diagnosis and treatment of low back pain: a joint clinical practice guideline from the American College of Physicians and the American Pain Society. Ann Intern Med 2007;147:478–91.

13. Dagenais S, Caro J, Haldeman S. A systematic review of low back pain cost of illness studies in the United States and internationally. Spine J 2008;8:8–20.

14. Yanni LM, McKinney-Ketchum JL, Harrington SB, et al. Preparation, confidence, and attitudes about chronic noncancer pain in graduate medical education. J Grad Med Educ 2010;2:260–8.

15. Chen J, Fagan M, Diaz J, et al. Is treating chronic pain torture. Internal medicine residents' experience with patients with chronic nonmalignant pain. Teach Learn Med 2007;19:101–5.

16. Upshur CC, Luckmann RS, Savageau JA. Primary care provider concerns about management of chronic pain in community clinic populations. J Gen Intern Med 2006;21:652–5.

17. Green CR, Wheeler JR, Marchant B, et al. Analysis of the physician variable in pain management. Pain Med 2001;2:317–27.

18. Barry DT, Irwin KS, Jones ES, et al. Opioids, chronic pain, and addiction in primary care. J Pain 2010;11:1442–50.

19. Turk DC, Swanson KS, Tunks ER. Psychological approaches in the treatment of chronic pain patients: when pills, scalpels, and needles are not enough. Can J Psychiatry 2008;53:213–23.

20. Turk DC, Okifuji A. Psychological factors in chronic pain: evolution and revolution. J Consult Clin Psychol 2002;70:678.

21. Pincus T, Burton AK, Vogel S, et al. A systematic review of psychological factors as predictors of chronicity/disability in prospective cohorts of low back pain. Spine 2002;27:E109–20.

22. Kerns RD, Sellinger J, Goodin BR. Psychological treatment of chronic pain. Annu Rev Clin Psychol 2011;7:411–34.

23. Morley S, Eccleston C, Williams A. Systematic review and meta-analysis of randomized controlled trials of cognitive behaviour therapy and behaviour therapy for chronic pain in adults, excluding headache. Pain 1999;80:1–13.

24. Hoffman BM, Papas RK, Chatkoff DK, et al. Meta-analysis of psychological interventions for chronic low back pain. Health Psychol 2007;26:1–9.
25. Sharpe L, Schrieber L. A blind randomized controlled trial of cognitive versus behavioral versus cognitive-behavioral therapy for patients with rheumatoid arthritis. Psychother Psychosom 2012;81:145–52.
26. Thorn BE, Day MA, Burns J, et al. Randomized trial of group cognitive behavioral therapy compared with a pain education control for low-literacy rural people with chronic pain. Pain 2011;152:2710–20.
27. Okie S. A flood of opioids, a rising tide of deaths. N Engl J Med 2010;363:1981–5.
28. CDC. CDC grand rounds: prescription drug overdoses—a U.S. epidemic. Available at: http://www.cdc.gov/mmwr/preview/mmwrhtml/mm6101a3.htm. Accessed July 3, 2012.
29. Boudreau D, Von Korff M, Rutter CM, et al. Trends in long-term opioid therapy for chronic non-cancer pain. Pharmacoepidemiol Drug Saf 2009;18:1166–75.
30. Braden JB, Sullivan MD, Ray GT, et al. Trends in long-term opioid therapy for non-cancer pain among persons with a history of depression. Gen Hosp Psychiatry 2009;31:564–70.
31. Edlund MJ, Steffick D, Hudson T, et al. Risk factors for clinically recognized opioid abuse and dependence among veterans using opioids for chronic non-cancer pain. PAIN 2007;129:355–62.
32. Becker WC, Sullivan LE, Tetrault JM, et al. Non-medical use, abuse and dependence on prescription opioids among US adults: psychiatric, medical and substance use correlates. Drug Alcohol Depend 2008;94:38–47.
33. SAMHSA. Substance Abuse and Mental Health Services Administration (2011). Results from the 2010 National Survey on Drug Use and Health: summary of national findings, NSDUH Series H-41, HHS Publication No. (SMA) 11–4658. Rockville (MD): Substance Abuse and Mental Health Services Administration; 2011.
34. Drug Abuse Warning Network. Amphetamine and methamphetamine emergency department visits, 1995-2002. Rockville (MD): Substance Abuse and Mental Health Services Administration; 2002.
35. Warner M, Chen L, Makuc D. Increase in fatal poisonings involving opioid analgesics in the United States, 1999-2006. NCHS data brief, no 22. Hyattsville (MD): National Center for Health Statistics; 2009.
36. Becker WC, Tobin DG, Fiellin DA. Nonmedical use of opioid analgesics obtained directly from physicians: prevalence and correlates. Arch Intern Med 2011;171:1034–6.
37. Starrels JL, Becker WC, Weiner MG, et al. Low use of opioid risk reduction strategies in primary care even for high risk patients with chronic pain. J Gen Intern Med 2011;9:958–64.
38. Martell BA, O'Connor PG, Kerns RD, et al. Systematic review: opioid treatment for chronic back pain: prevalence, efficacy, and association with addiction. Ann Intern Med 2007;146:116–27.
39. Fishbain DA, Cole B, Lewis J, et al. What percentage of chronic nonmalignant pain patients exposed to chronic opioid analgesic therapy develop abuse/addiction and/or aberrant drug-related behaviors? a structured evidence-based review. Pain Med 2008;9:444–59.
40. Turk DC, Swanson KS, Gatchel RJ. Predicting opioid misuse by chronic pain patients: a systematic review and literature synthesis. Clin J Pain 2008;24:497–508.
41. Chou R, Fanciullo GJ, Fine PG, et al. Clinical guidelines for the use of chronic opioid therapy in chronic noncancer pain. J Pain 2009;10:113–30.

42. O'Brien CP, Volkow N, Li T. What's in a word? Addiction versus dependence in DSM-V. Am J Psychiatry 2006;163:764–5.
43. Johnson RE, Jaffe JH, Fudala PJ. A controlled trial of buprenorphine treatment for opioid dependence. JAMA 1992;267:2750–5.
44. Johnson RE, Chutuape MA, Strain EC, et al. A comparison of levomethadyl acetate, buprenorphine, and methadone for opioid dependence. N Engl J Med 2000;343:1290–7.
45. Malinoff HL, Barkin RL, Wilson G. Sublingual buprenorphine is effective in the treatment of chronic pain syndrome. Am J Ther 2005;12(5):379–84.
46. Alford DP, Compton P, Samet JH. Acute pain management for patients receiving maintenance methadone or buprenorphine therapy. Ann Intern Med 2006;144: 127–34.
47. Blondell RD, Ashrafioun L, Dambra CM, et al. A clinical trial comparing tapering doses of buprenorphine with steady doses for chronic pain and co-existent opioid addiction. J Addict Med 2010;4:140.
48. Weiss RD, Potter JS, Fiellin DA, et al. Adjunctive counseling during brief and extended buprenorphine-naloxone treatment for prescription opioid dependence: a 2-phase randomized controlled trial. Arch Gen Psychiatry 2011;68:1238–46.

Bending the Cost Curve and Increasing Revenue

A Family Medicine Model that Works!

Bernard J. Katz, MD, MBA*, Mark R. Needham, MD, MBA

KEYWORDS

- Revenue • Cost • Profitability • Contracting • Practice enhancements

KEY POINTS

- Family physicians looking to expand services need to consider their expertise and interest in the multiple opportunities in the community in which they practice.
- It is imperative that practices develop an organizational culture focused on rigorous financial management and set aside dollars for capital for investment. Furthermore, it is important to understand space allocation opportunities, for example using the day space for a nighttime sleep study center, and to develop stimulating and rewarding roles and responsibilities for all staff members as well as provide protected time to devote to developing new skills.
- Understanding the competitive landscape in the surrounding area is important. The development of a highly functional practice that is able to bend the cost curve and increase revenues is not a short-term, turnkey proposition, Moreover, it is not necessarily feasible to try all of the suggestions presented in this article at the same time; rather, the practice needs to determine what works best given the marketplace, and focus on those areas.

As family physicians face increasing economic pressures with changes in insurance reimbursement from government and nongovernment payers coupled to economic hardships that many patients face such as unemployment and higher out-of-pocket expenses, it is important that practices look critically at the financial impact of both building and sustaining a primary care Patient Centered Medical Home. This article highlights lessons learned and key strategies used by a successful California Family Medicine practice. By incorporating new models and revisiting time-tested methods for enhancing practice revenues, this article is not intended to serve as

Relationships: Bernard J. Katz, MD has no relationships to disclose. Mark R. Needham, MD is a faculty member of the National Procedures Institute in Radiology.
University of California, Los Angeles, 6029 Bristol Parkway, Suite 100, Culver City, CA 90230, USA
* Corresponding author.
E-mail address: bjkatz@mednet.ucla.edu

a comprehensive list of "to dos" but rather to serve as a potential checklist to ensure maximum revenues.

PAYER AGREEMENTS: READ THE CONTRACT

Most family physicians act as participating providers in a variety of insurance plans. Although Medicare and Medicaid reimbursements are set by the government and are not open for negotiation, family physicians may be able to negotiate with some preferred provider organizations (PPOs), health maintenance organizations (HMOs), and independent practice associations (IPAs). Typically physicians enter into individual contracts with PPO plans. These contracts are sometimes received unsolicited, while at other times being requested by the physician. Typical supply and demand economics often apply to payer contracting. A contract received unsolicited may indicate that the payer is looking to grow its' primary care physician workforce, which may allow physicians who are negotiating from themselves or a group some leverage in setting rates.

It goes without saying that physicians need to carefully read the payer agreement.

Unfortunately and all too often, physicians simply sign and return a contract without reading and understanding all of the provisions, especially the information regarding renewal agreements. While the reimbursement rate is an important part of the agreement, it is important that every section of the contract is carefully analyzed and understood. Before negotiating a new or existing payer agreement contract, family physicians need to analyze the current state of their practice and determine if there are specific items of importance that need to be fully discussed before signing a payer agreement, whether new or existing.

LIST SERVICES PROVIDED AND SCOPE OF PRACTICE

Create a table of the scope of services offered by the practice. This table does not need to be exhaustive but should include practice locations such as office, hospital, and skilled nursing facilities. Furthermore, make a list of the frequently billed Current Procedural Terminology (CPT) codes by location, including codes for all procedures performed in all practice locations. The breadth of procedures offered will depend on the marketplace but may include office-based procedures such as colposcopy, laceration repair, treadmill testing, electrocardiograms, and so forth. In addition, some offices may offer imaging, Clinical Laboratory Improvement Amendments (CLIA)-waived laboratory services as well as hospital and outpatient surgery center billable services. Finally, list as an added value of your practice extended office hours, urgent care services, or any other services not usually provided in a "typical" family medicine practice (**Table 1**).

Create a snapshot of the practice contract renewal dates by payer, and determine the amount of reimbursement by payer and what percentage each payer contributes to the practice income (**Table 2**). It is important to recognize when a particular agreement will renew, as old rates may continue to prevail if newer rates are not negotiated.

Using the list of services from **Table 1**, create a "market basket" of typical CPT codes with the current reimbursement rates for the top 5 or 10 payers for the practice (**Table 3**). In **Table 3**, 3 payers (A–C) with 2 common CPT codes billed are the outpatient new and established patient-visit codes. The reimbursements by payer would be compared, and it would be determined whether the reimbursement rates were acceptable or that a particular contract agreement should not be continued without significant changes in reimbursement.

Table 1
A list of services not usually provided in a "typical" family medicine practice

Scope of Practice	Outpatient	Hospital	Skilled Nursing Facility	Office-Based				Extended Hours or Urgent Care	Hospital or Surgery Center
				Procedures	Imaging	Point-of-Care Testing	Vaccines and other biological agents		
List top 5–10 Payers	E&M codes	E&M codes	E&M codes						Assistant surgeon colonoscopist
Payer A	Most frequent CPT codes								
Payer B	Most frequent CPT codes								
Payer C	Most frequent CPT codes								

Table 2
Periodic practice review of payer contracts and percent of business by payer

| | | Date Reviewed | | |
Payer	Original Contract Date	Renewal/ Termination Date	Reimbursement by Payer ($)	% of Income by Payer
A	1/1/2012	12/31/2013	800,000.00	33%
B	—	—	—	—
C	—	—	—	—
D	—	—	—	—
E	—	—	—	—

IDENTIFY SPECIFIC NUANCES FOR EACH CONTRACT

Analyzing current payer agreements will help identify specific nuances in particular contracts. Important areas to focus on include (but are in no way limited to) the following:

1. How much time is allowed to submit a claim? For some payers, they limit submission to within 90 days of the date of service and will not pay a claim received after 90 days from date of service.
2. If a claim is rejected, how much time is available to resubmit and challenge the denial?
3. Does the payer specifically bundle certain services and disallow additional payment? Keep a watchful eye, as some payers may try to bundle in-office CLIA-waived point-of-care testing as part of the office visit.
4. Will the payer reimburse the family physician for all services that (s)he is able to perform? For example, will office-based treadmill testing performed by the family physician be paid or does the payer require that the patient have the test performed by a cardiologist?

Table 3
CPT code reimbursement by payer and location/activity

	Payer A Reimbursement ($)	Payer B Reimbursement ($)	Payer C Reimbursement ($)
New Outpatient Visit			
99205			
99204			
99203			
99202			
99201			
Subtotal A			
Established Outpatient Visit			
99215			
99214			
99213			
99212			
99211			
Subtotal B			

5. Does the payer provide additional compensation for services not usually provided in the normal scope of practice such as extended hours, house calls, and telephone or electronic mail consults? Having a practice operate an urgent care or offering extended office hours is advantageous for many payers, as it reduces the number of emergency room visits that are ultimately more costly for the majority of payers. It is important to keep in mind that family medicine practice incurs additional costs by remaining open after usual business hours. Although CPT codes do exist for the provision of extended office hours-based care (99050 and 99051), it is important to ask:
    a. Will the payer agree to pay for extended office hours?
    b. Will the payer reimburse for these codes 99050 and 99051 and modifiers, or will they bundle the payment and disallow any additional payment?
6. When the payer requests copies of records for use review, quality assurance, or payment queries, who is responsible for making the copies?
    a. Will the payer reimburse the practice for copies? If so, at what rate?
    b. Has a rate been established for paper records versus electronic records?
7. If the contract agreement terminates, how will the physician be paid after termination? Many payer agreements require that physicians continue to care for patients in the middle of treatment, such as hospital inpatients until the patient is discharged, even if the agreement terminates. If the physician is capitated, will additional payments be made on a fee-for-service basis?
8. How much notice is required to terminate the agreement? Review whether the agreement contains an "evergreen" clause. This clause allows for the automatic renewal for subsequent terms unless the physician actively terminates it. If it does contain such a clause, then how much notice does the physician need to provide? Some payer agreements may have a notice provision requiring up to 1 year's notice for the physician to terminate, but the payer may terminate with just 30 days' notice.
9. What form of notice to terminate an agreement is required? Carefully read the notice provision language. A notice of termination may not be valid if not performed exactly as specified in the "notice section" of the agreement.
10. If the practice bills as a group entity, will the payer allow new physicians to join the practice if requested by the practice as long as the physician meets credentialing requirements?
11. Does the payer allow for the provision of services by mid-level practitioners such as nurse practitioners and physician assistants? If so, what services and will reimbursement be made that the same rate as a physician or at a reduced rate?
12. Does the physician have the ability to elect to "close panel" and limit the acceptance of new patients? Is the practice able to do this only with respect to that particular payer, or is it tied to the practice being closed to new patients from any payer source?
13. Does the agreement include the ability for other payers to "piggy back" onto the agreement without the practice's consent? For example, the practice may agree to a contract based on the assumption that the patients will be from a particular employer, regional location, and so forth, only to find that other employers are able to use the payer's negotiated provider network and thus expand the number of potential patients that the practice sees at these negotiated rates. If the rates are favorable the practice should be agreeable to this. However, if the contract was viewed as a "loss leader" then this "silent PPO" issue may result in the practice seeing more patients at a reimbursement rate that is not favorable to the bottom line.

14. Does the agreement contain any exclusivity language whereby the payer attempts to limit the ability of the physician to join or contract with another group or payer?
15. Does the agreement have any nonsolicitation language limiting the ability of the physician to notify patients if a decision is made not to renew a particular agreement?

Although a particular practice may find that it needs to continue to contract with a particular payer and that it has little negotiating leverage with the payer, the practice will at least be aware of the specifics of the agreement.

PRACTICE ENHANCEMENTS

In the previous section, the importance of understanding contract agreements from a selective and informed position was presented. Increasingly there will be opportunities to develop innovative patient-centered medical home (PCMH) models that effectively use health information technology to drive clinical and business decisions as well as leverage contract negotiations with strategic community partners. Discussed here are strategies used by a 21-physician member practice in West Los Angeles. Although all of the practice enhancements used by this physician group may not fit all practice groups, exploring practice enhancements need to be part of any PCMH checklist. This section discusses office-based imaging, certified laboratory services, sleep medicine, procedural service lines, and the use of telephone and e-visits.

Imaging

There are several ways to increase revenue through imaging procedures. The most common is to perform radiography within the office practice. The cost of digital radiograph packages for office use has decreased, making it feasible for physicians even in solo practice to provide this service, and it is certainly a revenue booster for a practice of 4 or more physicians. Any practice skewed toward urgent care will find radiography probably essential for patient care, but definitely a revenue booster. Offering radiographs in the office will require hiring certified x-ray technologists as well as the supervising physician obtaining an x-ray supervisor license to be able to assure radiation safety. Physicians trained in reading radiographs can bill a global fee to provide the service. An alternative is for the primary care physician office to perform the radiography and bill for the technical component, and arrange for a radiologist to provide the reading and also bill for the professional component. Either arrangement will increase revenue for the primary care office.

Another radiology service that can be provided in the primary care office is bone densitometry. Although there are several low-cost bone density devices, such as those that measure bone density at the ankle, these may function at less than optimal reliability and reproducibility. The preferred method for providing bone density analysis is by DEXA, dual-energy x-ray bone absorptiometry. Unlike regular x-ray rooms, the examination room that houses the DEXA unit does not require lead shielding, as the radiation emitted during an examination is very low. Similar to having radiography services, the office will need a technician certified in DEXA to perform the examination and the physician must be trained in interpretation of the study. A group practice of 2 to 4 doctors would find the addition of DEXA screening to be a solid boost to practice revenue.

In recent years the cost of ultrasound units has come down, now making it realistic for primary care doctors to provide ultrasonography and echocardiography in their offices. A certified ultrasonography technician must be hired to perform the diagnostic tests, which may include gall bladder, renal, and pelvic scans as well as screening for aortic aneurysm and carotid artery stenosis. Many ultrasound units also can be configured for echocardiography. The physicians that choose to provide these imaging services must have special training to become proficient in the interpretation of these studies. Several organizations, including the National Procedures Institute, provide training in these modalities.

Beyond CLIA-Waived Point-of-Care Testing

Most offices provide CLIA-waived tests such as urinalysis. It is possible for group practices to provide more advanced laboratory testing, such as complete blood counts, chemistry panels, and some immunologic testing. Clinical laboratories such as this will require state licensing, periodic recredentialing, employment of certified laboratory technologists, enrollment in national proficiency testing programs, and rigorous oversight by the physician laboratory director, as there is significant liability associated with laboratory testing. However, a group practice of at least 6 busy physicians can support an in-office clinical laboratory, and the revenue from the laboratory will exceed the cost of the equipment, reagents, laboratory technicians, and regulatory oversight. For a busy group practice a laboratory can be an excellent revenue booster.

Sleep Medicine

For a group practice of at least 10 physicians, and one that includes a neurologist or pulmonologist interested in sleep medicine, an overnight sleep laboratory can be a good revenue booster. Ideally the sleep-study laboratory could be housed in the existing office space and converted to sleep-diagnostic beds at night. Obstructive sleep apnea is underdiagnosed and is often contributory or causative of other medical conditions diagnosed in the primary care office. In addition to the proper facility and equipment providing diagnostic sleep services, this service line will also require certified sleep technologists to administer the test and board-certified physicians to interpret the studies. However, revenue from the studies can be an excellent revenue booster for a practice, as these studies are periodically repeated to determine the appropriate settings for continuous positive airway pressure (CPAP) therapy. In some circumstances, the sale of durable medical equipment, such as the CPAP devices and masks, may add additional revenue to the practice.

Additional Service Lines

Cardiodiagnostics

Holter monitors and exercise treadmill testing require specialized equipment, but the equipment is not prohibitively expensive, even for a group practice of 2 to 4 physicians. The interpreting physicians must have training in these procedures, but once training is complete this will be a revenue booster, particularly if the practice is skewed toward older patients.

Endoscopy

A gastroenterology residency is not required to perform endoscopy and colonoscopy. However, additional training at special courses is required, and most endoscopy centers will require a primary care physician interested in performing these procedures to demonstrate training and to have a mentoring and supervision program in place before they become fully credentialed to perform the procedures independently. Although it is not an easy undertaking to accomplish the training and obtain credentialing privileges, these procedures are valuable to patients and can provide a significant revenue boost to the practice.

Telephone and e-visits
Traditional models of delivery of care are changing, and patients may request evaluation and management services outside of the traditional office setting. The practice should consider the use of telephone consults and e-visits to provide clinically appropriate services. Fees should be charged for providing these services, but it can be a challenge if insurers are bundling these services and consider them as part of the "primary care package." A secure network must be used to ensure the privacy and security of protected health information (PHI). Several commercially available software solutions exist for providing these services.

EVALUATE WORK FLOWS: WORK SMARTLY AND EFFICIENTLY

Personnel will typically be the largest variable expense in any primary care office. As office technology changes, such as implementing an electronic medical record or the office personnel becomes more experienced, it may be possible to make the office more efficient and reduce staff. Periodically a physician or group practice serious about keeping expenses down must perform a workflow analysis of the entire office. Several models exist that help the practice determine whether all of the steps in the process or flow are actually necessary or add any value to the operation, or might be possible to eliminate. For example, having a health team member screen calls to determine if an office visit is truly necessary may provide the physician with a sense of a protected schedule. However, if the practice recognizes that a patient's request for an appointment will most likely end up in an appointment being scheduled, at some point then it is better to just empower the front-office staff with scheduling an appointment when requested by a patient, without input from other unlicensed personnel. It is useful to ask members of the health care team how they think something could be done better or less expensively, and award bonuses to staff who offer successful ideas on expense reduction.

NEVER LOSE AN OPPORTUNITY WITH A PATIENT

Patients come to their family physician for advice and counseling. Tests are run and there is an obligation to notify patients of the results. While this can be done easily via telephone or mail, the best way is to schedule a visit with a patient to discuss the results in person, thus providing the family physician with adequate time to review the results, initiate changes in treatment if applicable, and discuss follow-up items that may be necessary. If results are completely normal then notifying the patient of the results may suffice and can be accomplished via mail, phone, or secure e-mail. However, many patients welcome the opportunity of scheduling a follow-up visit with their physician.

In addition, when patients are in the office, the workflow should ensure that the patient always stops at the checkout desk to not only make whatever payment may be owed for the visit but also to schedule a follow-up visit if suggested by the physician. Too many patients leave the office having been told to schedule a follow-up for medical reasons, only to never follow through on such an appointment. Patients will always have the opportunity to cancel the appointment if it is no longer necessary.

PHYSICIAN AND PATIENT TIME IS VALUABLE

Patients seek advice and medical consultation in a variety of ways. It is important that the physician's time is valued appropriately and that the physician and his or her team members also recognize that an hour lost can never be regained. Consider implementing some basic charges that alone will not enhance revenue significantly but will help to highlight the value of physician time and set practice expectations, including charges for:

1. Late cancellations. Consider charging patients for appointments not canceled within 24 hours' notice. A patient "no show" for an appointment has used up a slot that could have been used by another patient and that cannot be regained.
2. Telephone consultations using standard coding guidelines.
3. E-mail consultations using standard coding guidelines.
4. After-hours telephone consultation. Although the physician may not actually choose to bill the patient, it may cut down on call or e-mails that are able to be addressed the following business day.

BILLING FOR PROFESSIONAL SERVICES: MAKE SURE YOU ARE PAID FOR WHAT YOU DO!

It is discouraging when a physician's hard work is not ultimately rewarded by appropriate reimbursement. The effective practice will regularly review the performance of the billing and collections office. The entire revenue cycle must periodically be reviewed and audited. The practice must assess and be confident that all:

1. Charges are captured
2. Charge documents are delivered to the billing office
3. Charges are posted by the billing office or vendor
4. Charges are submitted for insurance payment on a timely basis
5. Patient balances are billed to the patient on a timely basis after action by the insurance company
6. Receipts are correctly entered
7. Cash is collected properly

In addition, the practice must periodically review the collections activity to ensure that outstanding balances are actively pursued, including requesting payment of outstanding balances at the front desk at the time that patients present for appointments, and to seek the maximum possible collections after contractual adjustments are factored in.

As previously discussed, contractual adjustments made by the payer need to be reviewed at least annually. It is important to select a sample of reimbursements by each payer and compare it with the terms contractually allowed and agreed on. The practice must seek accurate payments from insurance companies, and consider termination of contracts for those payers that fall to the bottom of the reimbursement list or fail to honor their contracts.

COLLECTING COPAYMENTS, PROMPT-PAY DISCOUNTS, AND INCENTIVE AWARDS

Encourage staff to collect copayment at the time of service and offer prompt-pay discounts. In addition, collect outstanding balances at the time of the visit. Often this requires that the clinical staff turn in the charge documents promptly and completely at the end of the visit. However, it is worth the time and effort it takes to do this so that the staff can assist with collections. In addition to collecting for any amounts due at the time of service, consider the following:

1. Charging for copayments not paid at the time of service. There is an expense incurred by the practice for balance billing, therefore it is reasonable to pass on a "billing fee" for copayments not paid at the time of service.

2. Providing a prompt-pay discount to uninsured patients who pay their discounted bill in full at the time of service. Billing fees are not incurred when full payment is made at the time of service, and the practice is more likely to be paid if payment is obtained at the time of service.
3. Providing a financial incentive to front-office staff to collect on old accounts. In some practices, it may be possible to share a portion of outstanding balances collected on old accounts. Consider providing incentive awards to the practice unit responsible for collecting on old accounts.

EXPENSE REDUCTION

In addition to reviewing the revenue received for services, it is important to also to analyze the expenses of the practice on a regular basis. Two significant expenses for the practice are the cost of labor and medical supplies.

Employee Costs

As previously noted, employee expenses are typically the most expensive variable expense in a family medicine practice. Periodic review of salaries in comparison with the marketplace is important. If the practice has regular staff turnover, any savings in lower salary expense will be offset in time spent training new employees and the adverse effect that this has on physician and practice productivity. Also, be sure that each member of the team is providing care in the most efficient way possible to ensure that physician time is not being spent on tasks that can be handled efficiently by other health care team members.

Supplies and Vendor Relationships

Medical supplies are typically the next most expensive variable expense. Family medicine practices frequently procure both biological and nonbiological medical supplies, frequently from the same vendor. The practice should set up regular meetings with the vendor to review purchasing patterns, products chosen, and potential discounts. Comparable products may be available at lower costs. For example, one practice delegated supply purchasing to a medical assistant who decided to always order latex-free examination gloves. These gloves are significantly more expensive than the regular "house-brand" gloves offered by the medical supplier. Changing to the regular house-brand gloves with a few boxes of latex-free gloves available for those patients with latex allergy resulted in a significant savings to the practice.

Some vendors may be willing to offer a discount either for volume or for a period of exclusivity. These agreements should be reviewed at least annually, to assure that the negotiated rates are being honored.

Biological medical supplies constitute a significant cost to family medicine practices. Use of generic agents may substantially reduce costs. In addition, meet with representatives of vaccine manufacturers and determine if savings can be obtained by using a particular vendor for most vaccines.

Group-Purchasing Organizations

Group-purchasing organizations (GPOs) may be available to a practice. These GPOs allow practices access to discounted rates for medical supplies, negotiated by the GPO with specific vendors. Sometimes GPOs are available through specialty societies or local physician organizations, whereas some are private companies. In some instances, a membership fee is required and many GPOs rebate savings to their members at the end of the year. The GPOs are positioned to negotiate markedly reduced rates, based on providing some exclusivity and volume purchasing to the manufacturer.

SUMMARY

As family physicians and other primary care physicians face the challenge of rising overheads and lower reimbursement rates, it is important to review opportunities to enhance revenue and streamline operations. Family physicians looking to expand services need to consider their expertise and interest in the multiple opportunities in the community where they practice.

It is imperative that practices develop an organizational culture focused on rigorous financial management and set aside dollars for capital for investment. Furthermore, it is important to understand space-allocation opportunities, for example using the day space for a nighttime sleep-study center, develop stimulating and rewarding roles and responsibilities for all staff members, and provide protected time to devote to developing new skills. Understanding the competitive landscape in the surrounding area is important. The development of a highly functional practice that is able to bend the cost curve and increase revenues is not a short-term, turnkey proposition, Moreover, it is not necessarily feasible to try all of the suggestions presented in this article at the same time; rather, the practice needs to determine what works best given the marketplace, and focus on those areas.

Index

Note: Page numbers of article titles are in **boldface** type.

A

Addiction
    behavioral medicine for, 607
    pain management and, 664–666
Affordable Care Act, 633–634, 646
Ambulatory care pharmacists, 617
American Academy of Family Physicians, patient-centered medical home definition of, 596–597
American Recovery and Reinvestment Act, 634
Anticoagulation clinic, family nurse practitioners in, 600
Anxiety, behavioral medicine for, 607
Assessment and Plan section, in electronic health record, 638–639
Auditing, electronic health record, 639–641

B

Back pain, management of, **661–669**
Behavioral medicine, **605–614**
    case example of, 610–611
    epidemiology of, 607–608
    for pain management, 663–664
    integration into practice
        case example of, 610–612
        preparation of, 608–609
        results of, 611–612
    rationale for, 606–607
Billing, 679
Bone densitometry, adding to practice, 676–677
Books, for self-management, 654
Brain waste, drain, and gain, in residence programs, 645

C

Cardiodiagnostics, adding to practice, 677
Centers for Medicare Services (CMS), 636–638, 641
Certification, for family nurse practitioner, 602
Change, motivation for, in self-management interventions, 650–651
Chief Complaint, in electronic health records, 636–637
Chronic Care Model, 597–599, 654
Chronic disease
    behavioral medicine in, **605–614**
    clinical pharmacists involvement in, **615–626**
    family nurse practitioners use in, **595–603**

Prim Care Clin Office Pract 39 (2012) 683–689
http://dx.doi.org/10.1016/S0095-4543(12)00092-9
0095-4543/12/$ – see front matter © 2012 Elsevier Inc. All rights reserved.

primarycare.theclinics.com

Chronic (*continued*)
  pain management for, **661–669**
  palliative care for, **627–631**
Claims, coding of, 636
Clinical information systems, in Chronic Care Model, 598–599 Clinical pharmacists,
  615–626
  barriers to implementation of, 620–622
  current status of, 617–618
  documentation for, 623
  education of, 616
  impact of, 616–617
  in patient-centered medical home model, 618–620
  recommendations for increasing use of, 623–624
  reimbursement models of, 622–623
Clinical Pharmacy Services Collaborative, 617
Cloning concept, in electronic health record, 634–639
Coaching sessions, for self-management, 655
Coding of claims, 636
Colonoscopy, adding to practice, 677
Communication, in self-management interventions, 652
Community resources and policies, in Chronic Care Model, 598
Competence, in self-management interventions, 653–654
Compliance audits, family nurse practitioners handling, 601
Contracts
  nuances in, 674–676
  understanding and negotiating, 672
Copayments, collecting, 679–680
Cost curve, bending of, for increasing revenue, **671–681**
Counseling, in electronic health record, 639
Current Procedural Terminology codes, 636, 672–673

  D

Daily reports, family nurse practitioners reviewing, 599
Decision support, in Chronic Care Model, 597–598
Decision-making, in electronic health record, 638–639
Delivery system design, in Chronic Care Model, 598
Depression, behavioral medicine for, 607
Diabetes Prevention Source Health's Behavior Change Suite, 655
Discounts, for prompt payment, 679–680
Disease management companies, for self-management, 655
Do not resuscitate orders, 628
Documentation
  electronic. *See* Electronic health record.
  for clinical pharmacy services, 623
  repetitive (cloning), 634–639
Drug knowledge, clinical pharmacists and. *See* Clinical pharmacists.

  E

Economic impact, of clinical pharmacists, 617
Education

in self-management interventions, 651
of clinical pharmacists, 616
of family nurse practitioners, 596
of international medical graduates, **643–648**
Efficiency, improving, 678
Electrocardiograms, family nurse practitioners reviewing, 599
Electronic health record
auditing of, 639–641
cloning in, 634–639
codlng of claims in, 636
inappropriate payments and, 636
medical decision-making in, 638–639
medical notes in, 635–636
quality problems in, 636–638
regulations for, 633–634
volume of documentation in, 635
E-mail visits, adding to practice, 678
Emotional regulation, in self-management interventions, 652
Employee costs, reduction of, 680
Endoscopy, adding to practice, 677
Environmental resources, for self-management interventions, 652–653
Examination, in electronic health record, 637–638
Expense reduction, 680–681

F

Family nurse practitioners, **595–603**
chronic care model and, 597–599
description of, 595–596
education for, 596
hiring, 602
in motivational interviewing, 601–602
in patient-centered medical home, 596–597
in travel medicine, 601
statistics on, 596
typical activities of, 599–601
Federal Documentation Guidelines, 638–639, 641
Follow-up visits, scheduling, 678

G

Group interventions, for self-management, 654
Group-purchasing organizations, 680–681

H

Health information technology, **633–642**
auditing in, 639–641
clinical pharmacists in, 618
cloning concept in, 634–639
coding of claims in, 636
inappropriate payments in, 636

Health (*continued*)
    medical decision-making in, 638–639
    quality issues in, 636–638, 641
    regulations affecting, 633–634
Health information Technology for Economic and Clinical Health Act, 634
Health Insurance Portability and Accountability Act (HIPAA), 633–634
History of Present Illness, in electronic health records, 636–637
Hospice care, versus palliative care, 627

I

Imaging, adding to practice, 676–677
Immigrant health care workers, **643–648**
Incentive awards, for collecting unpaid accounts, 679–680
Information systems, in Chronic Care Model, 598–599
Insurance
    contracts for, understanding and negotiating, 672
    reports and requests handling for, 601
International medical graduates, **643–648**
    impact of, 644–645
    laws concerning, 644
    linguistic barriers with, 645–646
    programs using, 646–647
Interviewing, motivational, family nurse practitioner in, 601–602

L

Lapses, coping with, in self-management interventions, 652
Linguistic problems, with international medical graduates, 645–646

M

Manuals, for self-management, 654
Media, for self-management, 654
Medical home. *See* Patient-centered medical home.
Medical Necessity
    documentation and, 635–636
    in electronic health record, 637
Medicare, documentation for, **633–642**
Medication prescriptions, family nurse practitioner responsibility for, 600, 602
Medication Therapy Management, 618
Mental health disorders, behavioral medicine for, 607
Migration, of medical graduates, **643–648**
Monitoring, in self-management interventions, 652
Motivation, in self-management interventions, 650–651
Motivational interviewing, family nurse practitioner in, 601–602

N

National Committee for Quality Assurance, patient-centered medical home definition of,
    596–597
National Survey on Drug Use and Health, 665
Nurse practitioners. *See* Family nurse practitioners.

O

Opioids, addiction to, pain management and, 664–666
Organizational support, in Chronic Care Model, 598

P

Pain management, **661–669**
    addiction and, 664–666
    behavioral medicine for, 608
    in palliative care, 627–631
Palliative care, in patient-centered medical home, **627–631**
Pap smears, abnormal, follow-up care in, 599
Patient-centered medical home
    behavioral medicine in, **605–614**
    clinical pharmacists in, 618–620
    economic issues in, **671–681**
    family nurse practitioner in, 596–597
    health information technology for, **633–642**
    international medical graduates in, 646
    pain management in, **661–669**
    palliative care in, **627–631**
    self-management interventions for, **649–660**
Pay for performance population, family nurse practitioners managing, 600–601
Payer agreements, understanding and negotiating, 672
Payments, inappropriate, 636
Pharmacists. *See* Clinical pharmacists.
Pharmacy e-Health Information Technology Collaborative, 618
Physician Orders for Life-sustaining Treatment document, 628
Physician Quality Reporting System, 634
Point-of-care testing, adding to practice, 677
Practice management
    behavioral medicine in, **605–614**
    clinical pharmacists in, **615–616**
    family nurse practitioners in, **595–603**
    health information technology in, 598–599, 618, **633–642**
    international graduates in, **643–648**
    pain management in, **661–669**
    palliative care in, **627–631**
    revenue enhancement in, **671–681**
    self-management interventions in, **649–660**
Prescriptions, family nurse practitioner responsibility for, 600, 602
Problem-solving, in self-management interventions, 652

Q

Quality
    family nurse practitioners in, 599–601
    in electronic health record, 636–638

R

Radiology, adding to practice, 676–677

Regulations
    of information systems, 633–634
    of pharmacist services, 618
Regulatory audits, family nurse practitioners handling, 601
Reimbursement
    billing for, 679
    for clinical pharmacy services, 622–623
Relieving Pain in America: A Blueprint for Transforming Prevention, Care and Education and Research, 662
Repetitive documentation (cloning), 634–639
Reports
    family nurse practitioners reviewing, 599
    insurance, 601
Residency programs, with international medical graduates, **643–648**
Revenue, increasing, **671–681**
    billing practices for, 679
    collecting copayments, discounts, and incentive awards for, 679–680
    expense reduction, 680–681
    facilitating follow-up visits for, 678
    identifying specific nuances for, 673–675
    list of services provided, 672–673
    payer agreements in, 672
    practice enhancements for, 676–678
    time management for, 678–679
    work flow evaluation for, 678
Review of Systems, in electronic health record, 635, 637

S

Safety, family nurse practitioners in, 599–601
Scope of practice, review of, 672–673
Self-directed Behavior, 654
Self-management interventions, **649–660**
    applying information in, 651
    as gold standard, 650
    competence development in, 653–654
    delivery vehicles for, 654–655
    elements of, 650–653
    environmental resources for, 652–653
    motivation for, 650–651
    skill development in, 651–652
    social support for, 653
Self-management support, in Chronic Care Model, 597
Services provided, list of, 672–673
Setbacks, coping with, in self-management interventions, 652
Skill development, in self-management interventions, 651–652
Sleep medicine, adding to practice, 677
Social support, in self-management interventions, 653
Stages of change model, 651
Stress management, in self-management interventions, 652
Substance abuse, behavioral medicine for, 607

Supplies, cost savings for, 680
Symptoms management, in palliative care, 627–631

T

Technology, for self-management, 655
Telephone consultation, adding to practice, 678
Time management, 678–679
Training. *See* Education.
Travel medicine, family nurse practitioner in, 601

U

Ultrasound, adding to practice, 676–677

V

Vendor relationships, cost savings in, 680

W

Wagner Chronic Care Model, nurse practitioner in, 597–599
Web sites, for self-management, 655
Work flow, evaluation of, 678

United States Postal Service
Statement of Ownership, Management, and Circulation
(All Periodicals Publications Except Requestor Publications)

1. Publication Title	2. Publication Number	3. Filing Date
Primary Care: Clinics in Office Practice	0 4 4 - 6 9 9 0	9/14/12

4. Issue Frequency	5. Number of Issues Published Annually	6. Annual Subscription Price
Mar, Jun, Sep, Dec	4	$216.00

7. Complete Mailing Address of Known Office of Publication (Not printer) (Street, city, county, state, and ZIP+4®)

Elsevier Inc.
360 Park Avenue South
New York, NY 10010-1710

Contact Person: Stephen R. Bushing
Telephone (Include area code): 215-239-3688

8. Complete Mailing Address of Headquarters or General Business Office of Publisher (Not printer)

Elsevier Inc., 360 Park Avenue South, New York, NY 10010-1710

9. Full Names and Complete Mailing Addresses of Publisher, Editor, and Managing Editor (Do not leave blank)

Publisher (Name and complete mailing address)

Kim Murphy, Elsevier, Inc., 1600 John F. Kennedy Blvd. Suite 1800, Philadelphia, PA 19103-2899

Editor (Name and complete mailing address)

Yonah Korngold, Elsevier, Inc., 1600 John F. Kennedy Blvd. Suite 1800, Philadelphia, PA 19103-2899

Managing Editor (Name and complete mailing address)

Barbara Cohen - Kligerman, Elsevier, Inc., 1600 John F. Kennedy Blvd. Suite 1800, Philadelphia, PA 19103-2895

10. Owner (Do not leave blank. If the publication is owned by a corporation, give the name and address of the corporation immediately followed by the names and addresses of all stockholders owning or holding 1 percent or more of the total amount of stock. If not owned by a corporation, give the names and addresses of the individual owners. If owned by a partnership or other unincorporated firm, give its name and address as well as those of each individual owner. If the publication is published by a nonprofit organization, give its name and address.)

Full Name	Complete Mailing Address
Wholly owned subsidiary of	1600 John F. Kennedy Blvd., Ste. 1800
Reed/Elsevier, US holdings	Philadelphia, PA 19103-2899

11. Known Bondholders, Mortgagees, and Other Security Holders Owning or Holding 1 Percent or More of Total Amount of Bonds, Mortgages, or Other Securities. If none, check box. ☑ None

Full Name	Complete Mailing Address
N/A	

12. Tax Status (For completion by nonprofit organizations authorized to mail at nonprofit rates) (Check one)
The purpose, function, and nonprofit status of this organization and the exempt status for federal income tax purposes:
☐ Has Not Changed During Preceding 12 Months
☐ Has Changed During Preceding 12 Months (Publisher must submit explanation of change with this statement)

PS Form 3526, September 2007 (Page 1 of 3 Instructions Page 3)) PSN 7530-01-000-9931 PRIVACY NOTICE: See our Privacy policy in www.usps.com

---

13. Publication Title	14. Issue Date for Circulation Data Below
Primary Care: Clinics in Office Practice	September 2012

15. Extent and Nature of Circulation		Average No. Copies Each Issue During Preceding 12 Months	No. Copies of Single Issue Published Nearest to Filing Date
a. Total Number of Copies (Net press run)		398	350
b. Paid Circulation (By Mail and Outside the Mail)	(1) Mailed Outside-County Paid Subscriptions Stated on PS Form 3541. (Include paid distribution above nominal rate, advertiser's proof copies, and exchange copies)	200	176
	(2) Mailed In-County Paid Subscriptions Stated on PS Form 3541 (Include paid distribution above nominal rate, advertiser's proof copies, and exchange copies)		
	(3) Paid Distribution Outside the Mails Including Sales Through Dealers and Carriers, Street Vendors, Counter Sales, and Other Paid Distribution Outside USPS®	38	40
	(4) Paid Distribution by Other Classes Mailed Through the USPS (e.g. First-Class Mail®)		
c. Total Paid Distribution (Sum of 15b (1), (2), (3), and (4))	▶	238	216
d. Free or Nominal Rate Distribution (By Mail and Outside the Mail)	(1) Free or Nominal Rate Outside-County Copies Included on PS Form 3541	60	69
	(2) Free or Nominal Rate In-County Copies Included on PS Form 3541		
	(3) Free or Nominal Rate Copies Mailed at Other Classes Through the USPS (e.g. First-Class Mail)		
	(4) Free or Nominal Rate Distribution Outside the Mail (Carriers or other means)		
e. Total Free or Nominal Rate Distribution (Sum of 15d (1), (2), (3) and (4))	▶	60	69
f. Total Distribution (Sum of 15c and 15e)	▶	298	285
g. Copies not Distributed (See instructions to publishers #4 (page 43))	▶	100	65
h. Total (Sum of 15f and g)	▶	398	350
i. Percent Paid (15c divided by 15f times 100)		79.87%	75.79%

16. Publication of Statement of Ownership

If the publication is a general publication, publication of this statement is required. Will be printed ☑ Publication not required
in the December 2012 issue of this publication.

17. Signature and Title of Editor, Publisher, Business Manager, or Owner

Stephen R. Bushing

Stephen R. Bushing –Inventory Distribution Coordinator

Date: September 14, 2012

I certify that all information furnished on this form is true and complete. I understand that anyone who furnishes false or misleading information on this form or who omits material or information requested on the form may be subject to criminal sanctions (including fines and imprisonment) and/or civil sanctions (including civil penalties).

PS Form 3526, September 2007 (Page 2 of 3)

Printed and bound by CPI Group (UK) Ltd, Croydon, CR0 4YY

13/10/2024

01773515-0001